Stretching
for
Beginners

Tips and Tricks to Some of the Best Stretching Methods to Improve Flexibility and Avoid Injuries

Emma Carter

Table of Contents

Introduction

Life today has become easier and more convenient, what with all the technological advancements that we get to enjoy. However, the convenience of modern living brings multiple stresses that tend to take a toll on our body and overall health. It could be from overwork, excessive use of technology, extreme sports play, or even being in a job that requires you to be sitting all day or constantly on the move.

Stress can cause the body to suffer from muscle pain and soreness, pinched nerves, and even more permanent disabilities, like severe body injuries. A quick, safe, and effective way to deal with such symptoms is stretching. The good thing about this simple therapy is that you can do it anytime and anywhere. Also, stretching does not require any special equipment.

If you want to learn more about stretching, its underlying principles, and how it can improve your flexibility, then you can use this book. In this comprehensive reading material, you can delve even deeper into what stretching and flexibility are all about and how to do stretches safely even if you are a beginner. It even tackles the technical and clinical aspects of stretching and flexibility in a simple and straightforward manner, so you can grasp them easily.

With that, expect to have an easier time understanding even those otherwise difficult concepts to grasp. Get well-rounded information about stretching for beginners and how you can use it to repair your body by getting a copy of this book. You will also learn how to use stretching exercises to make your body fitter, more relaxed, and flexible, and how to stretch safely as a senior.

Chapter 1

Stretching and Its Different Types

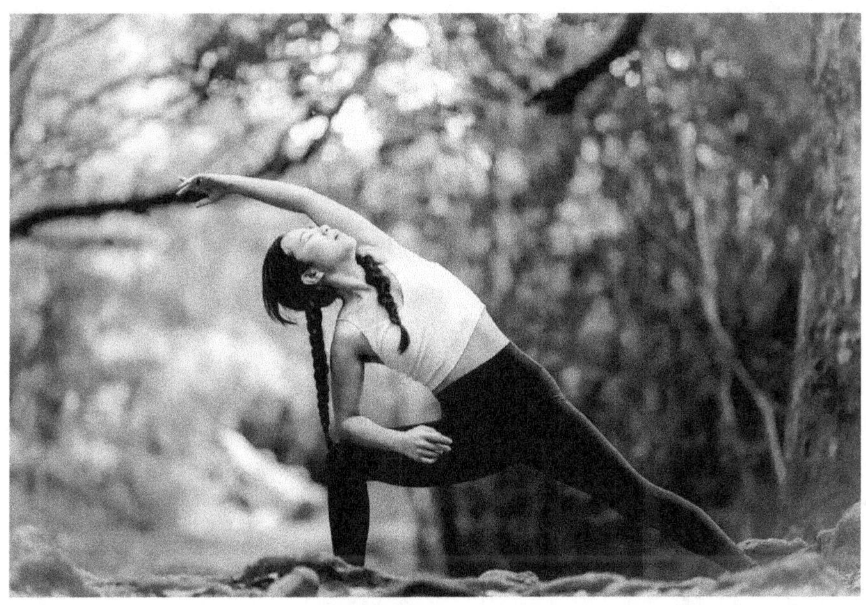

If you think that stretching is only for athletes, like gymnasts and runners, then you are wrong. It is an activity that everyone should do. Everyone needs to stretch as a means of protecting their mobility and health. Note that building muscles and attaining superior aerobic fitness is not usually enough to attain better health and fitness. It is also necessary to think about your flexibility, and you can only achieve that by stretching regularly.

Many people are unaware of how important it is to stretch regularly, but it is time to spread the information regarding how important it is to make it a part of your fitness routine. Stretching even needs to be a daily activity. It is what you need to keep your body flexible and mobile.

A Clearer Definition of Stretching

Stretching is a type of physical exercise that involves intentionally flexing or stretching a certain tendon, muscle, or muscle group as a means of boosting the elasticity of your muscles and attaining a more comfortable muscle tone. This results in increased flexibility, range of motion, and muscle control.

You can also use stretching therapeutically to help alleviate cramps. It can significantly improve your ability to function well when performing your daily activities.

As far as its basic form is concerned, you can look at stretching as an instinctive and natural activity. Humans are not the only ones who perform it. A lot of animals stretch, too. In most cases, this activity comes with yawning. Stretching happens by instinct, usually upon waking up from sleep, after leaving a confined area or space, or after being inactive for a prolonged period.

In terms of physical fitness, stretching is a basic tenet as it is the key to improving your flexibility. Athletes even make stretching a part of their routines. They use it to warm up before exercise and cool down right after. By doing that, they can lower their risk of dealing with injuries and boost their performance.

The Consequences of Inadequate Stretching

Stretching is a crucial aspect of your physical fitness as a lack of this physical exercise may lead to several issues that affect your body. For instance, not stretching enough can cause shortened muscles that can eventually develop painful knots.

Inadequate stretching can also make you prone to injury because you are not performing an activity designed to elongate your muscles. Poor flexibility caused by inadequate stretching may also negatively affect your joints.

It can lead to poor joint health as the joints need constant movement to keep up the health of your cartilage and the other structures within them. It is also the wide range of movements in your joints that can help in boosting blood supply and nutrients.

Another possible consequence of inadequate stretching is inflexible muscles that tend to tire out too quickly. When your muscles get tired easily, your opposing muscle groups will have to work doubly hard. This can further result in muscle fatigue and injuries.

When that happens, your muscles will also be unable to give your joints enough protection from chronic injuries. Your hamstrings, for instance, can contribute a lot to stabilizing your knees. It can also help prevent ACL tears.

One more thing that reduced flexibility brought on by inadequate stretching does is produce abnormal stress on every distant tissue and structure from the original site of inflexibility. A great example is knee tendonitis that also relates to tightness in the calf.

Muscles stretched regularly also have the advantage of enjoying better oxygenation, which may not happen if your muscles are tense. Having tense muscles mean they will be unable to receive enough vital nutrients and oxygen.

If you want to avoid the consequences of inadequate stretching, make it a habit to stretch before and after working out. By stretching before your workouts, your muscles will be prepared to receive the full impact of your exercise. Stretching after the exercise is also beneficial as it relaxes your muscles and prevents soreness.

Before working out, do some dynamic stretches like glute bridges and walking lunges. Static stretches that individually target certain muscles are also ideal for your cool-down exercises. Let's get to know more about these types of stretches in the next section.

Types of Stretching

Stretching comes in different types – with each stretch having its own benefits. Stretches can either be static (without motion) and dynamic (with motion). It is also further subdivided into other types that will allow you to pick the specific stretching techniques that produce the exact results you want.

Static Stretching

Static stretching is probably the most common among the different stretching types and techniques generally known. It often requires you to hold a stretch for around thirty to forty-five seconds with a short period of tension and a slow release. It is also further divided into two sub-types.

- **Active Stretching**, which involves only your body – In active stretching, you contract a muscle group to tense the opposing muscle group. One way to do this is to contract your hamstring as a means of stretching your quadriceps. Active stretching is your regular daily stretch.

- **Passive Stretching**, which requires the use of an external force or aid – This aid may come in the form of a stretching band or a wall. You may also seek the help of a partner. You can view passive stretching as more of an assisted form rather than the do-it-your-own approach.

Passive stretching can provide a dramatic improvement in your range of motion and flexibility. However, be careful when doing passive stretches as there are instances when it can result in overextension, leading to injuries.

Overall, static stretching has the advantage of increasing and expanding your flexibility and range of motion if you do it correctly. The most important aspect here is consistency and duration. It is recommended that you stretch at least 5 time a week for 5 minutes or more to benefit from having a better range of motion.

Dynamic Stretching

Dynamic stretching is all about stretching during warmups. It requires you to use deliberate movements designed to make your muscles lose as you warm them up and prepare them for physical activities. It also requires you to move in and out of a certain stretch. Think of the whole approach as an activity that is like accelerated yoga.

Dynamic stretching is mainly based on movements, which is why it is more popular among physical therapists and athletes. They view it as the ideal form of pre-exercise activity as it warms up muscles while preparing them for exertion.

This type of stretching also enhances your flexibility and range of motion while lowering your risk of injury caused by overextension. It can prevent muscle stiffness or excessive muscle looseness. What makes it even better is that it can reduce stiffness significantly right after completing the stretches.

Ballistic Stretching

Many confuse dynamic and ballistic stretching because the two are quite similar. However, ballistic stretching is different from dynamic stretching in the sense that it tends to incorporate highly intensive movement patterns into a stretch routine prior to an exercise.

Another difference is that ballistic stretching requires strong and fast muscle counter-movements that usually go over the typical range of movement. Therefore, it is not highly recommended for anyone who does not have any supervision from an expert.

One thing that ballistic stretching can do for the body is that it can help reduce the tightness in the muscles and tendons. However, it also involves high velocity, which may increase one's risk of injuring tendons and muscles, so whether it is good for the health and fitness of non-athletes or not is debatable.

However, while, it can relax your muscles and improve joint mobility, several experts still agree that it is not as beneficial as controlled dynamic and static stretching.

Isometric Stretching

Isometric stretching can be considered as a form of static stretching. In this stretching method, you will have to contract your muscles for a long period while you push against a form of resistance. Many of those who practice isometric stretching say it is more effective than passive or active stretching alone. The reason is that it can also strengthen your muscles.

Moreover, it is good for athletes who intend to achieve explosive power and speed whenever they engage their muscle group resistance. When performing isometric stretching, it is possible to utilize your body. You can also look for a partner who will be the one to apply resistance whenever you stretch.

Alternatively, you can utilize a form of resistance that comes from an external source. Some examples are gym equipment, floors, and walls. One way to do isometric stretching is to push against a wall so you can execute a calf stretch.

A single session of this form of stretching is tough and demanding on your muscles. That said, avoid making the mistake of training a single muscle group several times in a day with isometric stretching. Provided you do them correctly, some of the safest isometric stretches are calf raises, squats, plank, lunges, lateral raises, and wall sits.

Proprioceptive Neuromuscular Facilitation (PNF) Stretching

PNF is a combination of isometric and passive stretching, aimed at improve static-passive flexibility faster than other stretches when performed on their own. If you decide to do a PNF stretch, it would be best to begin with your muscle already in a contracted stretch. You should then move to the passive stretch. This procedure works in training your stretch receptors so they can get into a more improved and increased range of motion.

Initially designed to help rehabilitate stroke victims, PNF stretching is also used to treat sports injuries. You can do it with a partner or an expert, such as a physical therapist who will act as the external force while guiding your limb through its range of motion. A PNF stretching session consists of three phases.

- Passive stretching of the target muscle group

- Application of external force or resistance to attain an isometric contraction

- Relieved resistance together with the passive stretching of the muscle group again – In this phase, the range of motion should be greater. The practice is called post-isometric relaxation that the Golgi tendon organs found within your muscles tend to control.

A popular PNF stretching technique is the hold-relax. Other typical techniques in this stretching category are the hold-relax bounce, hold-relax-swing, rhythmic initiation, and contract-relax.

Myofascial Release

A myofascial release is a form of stretching exercise that involves using a foam roller or any other similar device. It is a hands-on stretching therapy designed to get rid of pain while restoring range of movement. It can offer relief from and help make your fascia, a specialized and densely woven system composed of connective tissues covering and uniting the compartments of your body, more flexible. It can also improve the flexibility of the underlying muscles.

In most cases, you can use myofascial release along with other therapies designed to treat muscular trauma, post-surgical stiffness, and pain, as well as inflammation. It is all about performing small and continuous movements over a certain area, around two to six inches, for 30 to 60 seconds. Your pain tolerance will have a say on the pressure level that you apply to the targeted area.

Overall, it may appear as a form of massage, but stretching involves the release of your myofascial tissue, which refers to a fibrous connective tissue composed of collagen supporting your bones and muscles. It helps those who are suffering from neck, back, and joint pain and those with myofascial pain syndrome or fibromyalgia. You can also find several myofascial release stretches that are safe to do at home without putting you at risk of injury.

Loaded Progressive Stretching

This type of stretching can help increase your range of motion using a load or external force. The load we are talking about here can be anything, like your own body weight, a barbell, or a dumbbell. You can start loaded progressive stretching with easy and simple static stretching poses. You then integrate a form of load to push your body to the point that it goes beyond the range of motion that it is comfortable with.

It is also possible to perform this stretching technique with a partner. One example is having your partner push on your back as you are in a seated pose with both your legs stretched out. Alternatively, you can integrate force by putting some sort of weight on your back. By integrating more weight or letting a partner push you harder whenever you do subsequent stretches, you can make that progressive component work.

Loaded progressive stretching is also a fantastic way to build stronger muscles. It allows you to stretch a lot deeper and hold poses longer. Make sure that you warm up and condition yourself before doing this stretching exercise, though. Also, it is recommended to start this exercise using low weights and several reps. That way, the stretches will be even more effective and intense.

Some of the most common types of stretching covered in this first chapter will be discussed again in detail later in the book, along with examples of exercises and routines that fall under them.

Chapter 2

Mobility vs. Flexibility: Is There a Difference Between the Two?

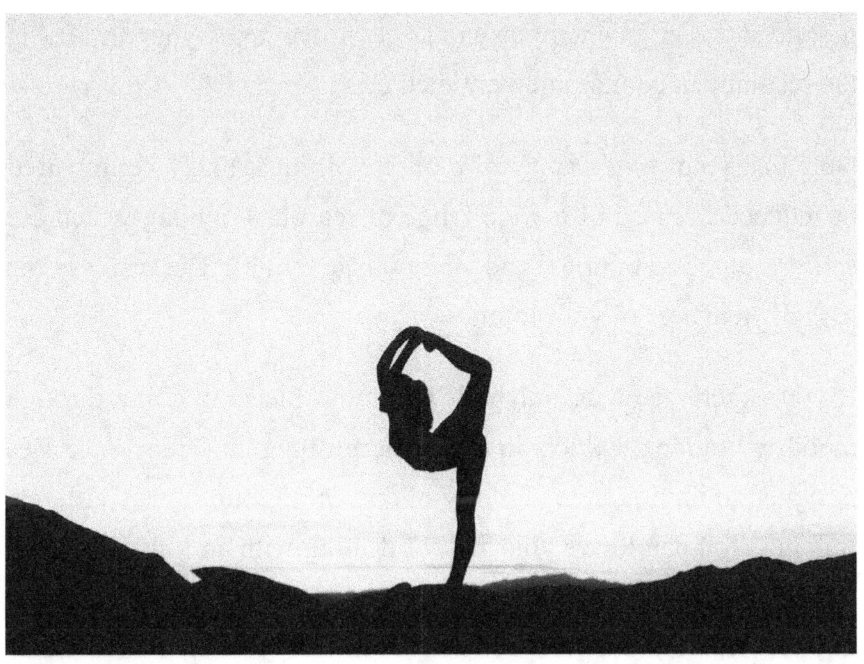

As explained, the main two aspects that stretching improves in your overall body, physique, and wellness are mobility and flexibility. Now the question is, are these two the same? Let's find out in this chapter.

Mobility Defined

Mobility refers to your ability to move your limbs using a wide range of movements. You can look at it as a controlled voluntary movement that involves going through the whole functional range of motion.

If you still have no idea about your level of mobility, you can measure it by standing straight than trying to rotate your shoulder. Raise your arm and move it back to the point that you can fully extend your arm straight beyond your head. A sign that you have a mobile shoulder is when you can freely move it and your arm using the recommended measurement method.

Note that your joint's range of motion will most likely be impaired or reduced because of a wide range of reasons – among which are sports exercises, injuries, and strenuous activities. The result is the overall weakness of your joints.

If you experience that, maybe it is time to focus on going through mobility training, which involves performing different exercises designed to improve the mobility of one or all your joints. With this training, you can lower your risk of dealing with an imbalance that may also subsequently result in you becoming less vulnerable to injuries. It can support better movements for sports or daily activities.

Mobility is vital for the overall quality of your life, especially as you age. By improving your mobility, you get the chance to move without any restrictions and pain. This results in you comfortably going through your everyday life, making it possible for you to execute a wide range of activities without any hassle.

To improve your mobility, you may want to include the following in your training plan.

- **Stretching** – It could be a static or the dynamic form of stretching. Regardless of what type of stretching you choose, it will help loosen up any tight and stiff muscles that may have stopped you from making certain movements.

  A dynamic stretch prior to every workout session, for instance, can prime your muscles and prepare them for the activity. An effective static stretch after your workout also has the advantage of alleviating any pain and soreness in your muscles.

- **Mobility Drills** – Choose mobility drills directed towards improving your range of motion. They should cover everything from relaxing, moving, and contracting your muscles. You can also isolate them to target certain areas or let them target several areas simultaneously.

- **Coordination** - Your training plan should also focus on improving your coordination. This is necessary for ensuring that your body will respond based on the way you want it to. Improving the coordination of your muscles and joints can help boost your performance while increasing your awareness of the positive effects of the training.

- **Balance** – You may also want to perform exercises that aim to improve your balance. This is important as it can improve your stability, thereby creating a solid foundation designed to give you an excellent base for your training. Among the best activities that will give you balance are Pilates and yoga.

- **Massage Techniques** – You may also want to employ some massage techniques to boost your mobility. In this case, you can use a massage ball, massage gun, or foam roller as a means of releasing your tight muscles.

It is also the key to lengthening them, thereby relieving you from pain. You may also want to get a professional massage now and then, as your therapist already knows the exact spot to target when trying to boost your performance.

Flexibility Defined

In terms of definition, flexibility differs from mobility because it basically refers to the lengthening ability of your muscles and your tendons and ligaments. It is your flexibility that makes it possible for your connective tissues to elongate temporarily. It is not the same as mobility since flexibility is more of a passive action.

Moreover, you can improve your flexibility through stretching. Note, though, that you do not necessarily have to stretch for hours on end to boost your flexibility. You can just dedicate a few minutes each day for stretching exercises capable of improving your body's range of motion.

Flexibility also refers to the ability to bend with ease and without breaking. It allows a particular movement to occur passively, giving you the chance to hold a specific stretch without causing pain in the targeted and surroundings joints.

Note that flexibility ranges differ from one person to another, because people also differ in terms of muscle length. You can improve it through regular stretching and exercise.

Relationship between Mobility and Flexibility

Both flexibility and mobility are vital for the overall quality of your life, especially as you age. The two can lower your risk of dealing with injuries and imbalance. Also, while it is the goal of many to improve their mobility, their quality of life, and their sports and physical activities, it is still your flexibility that you must address first.

You need to improve your flexibility before anything else as it is the function that can also subsequently lead to the improvement of your mobility. Your muscles need adequate flexibility to achieve sport-specific and functional mobility. This makes the two closely related since you need to work on your flexibility and mobility to achieve a better quality of life.

As mentioned, flexibility is considered as a passive activity. It refers to the ability to move your connective tissues using gravity, a tool, or another person. Your muscles will be the ones that will let the movements happen, though they must do it passively.

In most cases, you will experience some limitations in your flexibility because of a couple of structural issues.

- Tight and shortened tissues, including the muscles, ligaments, joint capsule, or fascia, resulting in joint movement restrictions

- Passive tissue degeneration, like the cartilage and the menisci or bony adaptations capable of blocking the proper movement of your joints

Any of the problems mentioned may cause some restrictions in your flexibility and your mobility. If your limitation is in hip flexibility, and you decide to do some hip mobility exercises, such as the lunge or overhead reach, it may not provide you with the gains and benefits you are hoping for.

The reason is that the mobility exercise does not address or target the main cause of the restriction, which is often purely structural. In the presence of flexibility limitations, you will also subsequently experience mobility restrictions. For instance, if you can't bend passively to 90 degrees, it would be impossible for you to bend to 90 degrees actively.

You can look at flexibility as a rubber band that stretches every time you pull both ends. The rubber is flexible because you can stretch it. In case it does not stretch, it is no longer flexible. The problem is if it becomes too inflexible, there is a high possibility that it will snap. This premise is also applicable to your muscles.

The elastic components in your muscles are designed to make moving through stretches possible.

Flexibility also needs your joint capsule to have a complete range of motion. Even if you have stretchy and flexible muscles, it will still not matter if your joints do not permit such movements. Because your mobility encompasses movements through a complete range of motion, it is crucial to incorporate flexibility stretches to help your muscles stay mobile.

With that said, you must not underestimate the importance of clearing your structural and flexibility issues before you work on improving your neuromuscular or mobility issues. Remember that mobility exercises can't repair all the issues that also tend to restrict your flexibility.

Better Mobility for Better Movements

Despite the close relationship between mobility and flexibility, it will become a problem if you think that flexibility alone is enough to improve your mobility. Yes, being flexible makes it possible for you to stretch your body into every position imaginable. This clearly indicates that your muscles have finally achieved superior flexibility, but the question is, are they controllable?

Having excellent mobility will let you execute several movement patterns without any restrictions. You can expect these movements to be efficient without any compensation. This will allow you to have an extensive range of motion, superior neuromuscular strength, and control that will let you move freely through a pattern.

Conversely, some can successfully execute a movement pattern, but they tend to compensate. They may fire a few muscles in various sequences, utilize various muscles to gain stability, or avoid specific joint positions.

This means that even if you are flexible, it is still possible for you to have or not have the stabilizer balance, coordination, or strength necessary in performing similar functional movements that someone with excellent mobility can do. This can then give you a clear idea of how fundamentally different flexibility and mobility are despite the close relationship between them.

Improving Your Mobility

Mobility is vital, and flexibility plays a crucial role in that. It does not necessarily mean you have to dedicate long hours in the gym to stretch and improve your flexibility, then subsequently, your mobility. You can just incorporate a steady flow of exercises that target the improvement of both your flexibility and mobility into your daily routines.

Aside from following a general approach, it also helps to dedicate some time to specific areas. By now, you are probably aware of the specific body parts and areas that you require improvement in. It could also be specific to the sports you are currently focusing on. If possible, seek the help of a professional as it can help you determine the specific areas to target and prioritize.

Apart from stretching and mobility drills, you can also spend some time doing dynamic warm-ups. It could be just 5 minutes or 30 minutes. This form of warm-up is effective in increasing your blood and muscle temperature and incorporating all the required movements necessary for your flexibility and mobility.

How about Range of Motion?

Another term that often goes hand in hand with flexibility and mobility is the range of motion (ROM). Note, though, that ROM also has its own meaning. Basically, it encompasses how far you can stretch or move a certain body part, like a muscle or joint.

ROM is different from one person to another. For instance, some can perform complete splits while others can't. Some can't do it because they have joints that are not loose enough and muscles that will not lengthen as far as necessary for the movement.

ROM, therefore, is the direction and distance through which your joints can move. Every joint comes with a standard ROM expressed in degrees. In physical therapy, the most common form of measurement used in measuring the total amount of motion available at a particular joint is known as goniometry. The ROM of a certain joint may have restrictions based on the articulating surfaces' shape and the ligamentous and capsular structures surrounding it.

You have a much better chance of improving your overall well-being and preventing injuries if you know what your ROM is exactly. It is also important for you to familiarize yourself with the two types of range of motion.

Active Range of Motion

A ROM refers to the space wherein you can move a specific body part with the help of your muscles. Here, you are exerting some effort without the help of any outside factors. For instance, if you lift your arms over your head as a means of stretching your muscles, such activity happens as part of your active ROM.

Passive Range of Motion

A passive ROM refers to the space wherein a specific body part can move with the help of something or someone who creates the movement. It could be through the help of a physical therapist or a massage. It is not you who engages the specific muscles that you typically use when starting the movement. In other words, you are seeking the help of an external factor that could be a person or thing.

Overall, your flexibility, mobility, and range of motion will be targeted by a wide range of stretching exercises. This means that the goal of stretching regularly recommended by experts is to help improve those three aspects of your physique and wellness.

By improving those, you will notice a huge improvement in your quality of life and overall health and fitness. Developing your flexibility, mobility, and range of motion can give you the freedom of movement designed to make your life worth living.

Chapter 3

Importance of Stretching and Flexibility Training

With the information that we have already presented in the previous couple of chapters, it is safe to say that stretching and flexibility training can contribute a lot to your health and fitness. If you struggle to touch your toes or deal with stiffness that limits your movements and your ability to perform your daily tasks, then maybe it is time to start integrating some stretching exercises in your routines and undergo flexibility training. It is time to stop overlooking the importance of flexibility training as it is truly a vital health-related element of your overall well-being.

Should You Make Stretching and Flexibility Training a Part of Your Life?

The answer is yes. The following are just some viable reasons why it is so important to make stretching and flexibility training a part of your daily life.

Lowers Stress

Chronic stress can trigger many undesirable body responses – among which are fatigue, tension, and anxiety. By stretching regularly, you can lessen the tension in your muscles. You can also combine it with mindful breathing to further lower your stress levels that may be causing your chronic anxiety and severe depression.

Promotes Better Posture

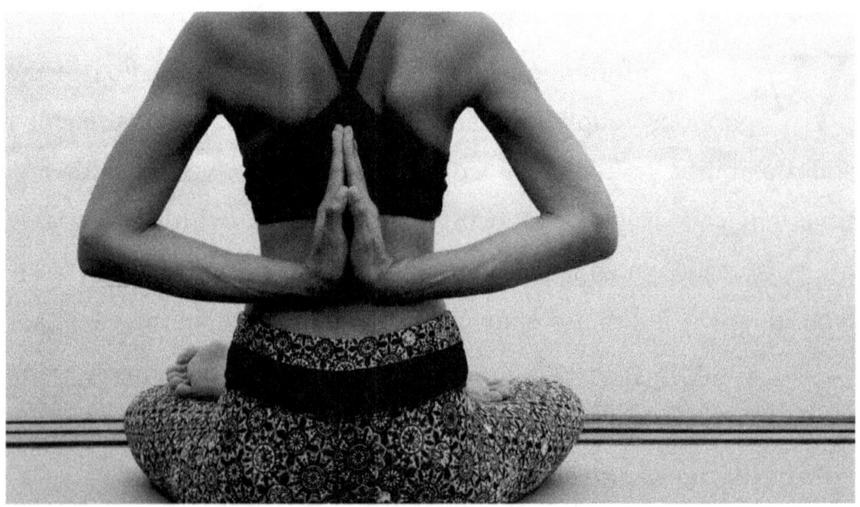

You may be tempted to skip your stretching routines now and then, but its benefits on your posture should give you the encouragement you need to try sticking with the training. Stretching can improve your posture in the sense that it can prevent your muscles from getting too tight. The result is your ability to maintain good posture even for an extended period.

The good thing about improving your posture is that it can lower your body's discomfort. It can even help reduce body pains and aches since you are able to stand and sit correctly. This can further lead to a significant improvement in your confidence and mood.

Controls Lower Back Pain

Frequent stretching and flexibility training also contribute to stronger lower back muscles. It can alleviate pain and soreness in the area. Constant stretching also keeps back pain brought on by constantly lifting heavy objects under control.

Reduces Stiffness and Pain

Excessive muscle tension can make your entire body increasingly uncomfortable. Static stretching exercises can particularly lower your pain levels as well as the stiffness of your muscles. It can also reduce the severity and frequency of muscle cramps. This results in you experiencing more comfort and minimal pains and aches.

Keeps Your Glutes Active

If you sit behind a desk the entire day, then you are at risk of giving your body an extremely hard time. Note that prolonged sitting, especially for several hours continuously in a day, can overexert your body, most especially your glutes.

Prolonged sitting may cause the shutdown of the nerves activating your glutes. Therefore, sitting a lot will put your glute muscles at risk of being in atrophy, meaning they will waste because of muscle degeneration.

Once your glutes shut down, it is highly likely that the joints and muscles surrounding them will become overstressed. The result is pains, aches, and stiffness, particularly those affecting your lower back.

To fight this negative effect, make it a point to activate your glutes. Get up from your seat, then stretch not only your glutes but also your hip flexors. Frequent stretching helps in reducing pain and injury in the future.

Improves Your Function

Certain factors like poor posture, improper body mechanics, prolonged sitting, and repetitive movement patterns can cause your body muscles to become chronically tight and tense. They may also contract. This leads to a significant reduction in their strength and suppleness that can affect your bodily function.

By stretching regularly and performing a wide range of flexibility training techniques, you can improve your overall function. You can achieve that benefit as your body will become even more effective in responding to the stresses that various activities and forms of movement impose.

It can also help enhance your performance as you will have better agility, muscular strength, power, and speed if you consistently include flexibility training and dynamic stretching into your fitness routines.

Makes You Less Prone to Injury

Another viable reason why you should make a habit out of stretching and take part in flexibility training is that it significantly contributes to lowering your risk of suffering from injuries. Dynamic stretches, for instance, can form part of your warm-up exercises as they can help raise your core body temperature while functionally preparing your body for the upcoming movements.

This makes stretching a vital component in preventing injuries. Through your regular stretches before any strenuous physical activity or sports, your body's tendons and cold muscles will have a lower chance of experiencing strains, sprains, and ruptures.

Improves Blood Circulation and Flow

Many consider improved blood circulation and flow as an essential benefit of stretching and flexibility as far as your health and wellness are concerned. Various stretching activities can increase and boost your circulation. Note that while stretching may not be capable of directly preventing injuries from excessive use, it is effective when it comes to increasing blood flow and supplying your muscles and cartilage with a wide range of essential nutrients.

This activity can significantly improve blood circulation and flow, contributing to the enhanced transportation of nutrient-rich blood and oxygen throughout your entire body. With the help of your stretching and flexibility exercises, you can also prevent your muscles from getting sore after your workout. This can further lead to minimal pain and dramatic improvements in your daily routines and activities.

Improves Sleep and Mood

Stretching also has a very relaxing effect, which can translate to better sleep and mood. Note that tight muscles may only cause your body to experience extreme stress. This can significantly hamper your sleep and mood. Undue stress even has an impact on you both physically and emotionally.

If you stretch, you are allowing yourself to let go. The kind of release you will be getting as you do your stretching exercises gives you the chance to connect yourself to your own body. It can also contribute to clearing your mind and purging all negative energies you are experiencing. This is a good thing as it can also give you a positive mood.

Apart from mental clarity and instant relief from stress, stretching can also improve your sleep. Regular morning stretches combined with light exercises are more effective in giving you a sound sleep than other exercises and activities.

Better Muscle Coordination

Stretching can also result in better muscle coordination. You can expect this activity to produce substantial improvements in your neuromuscular coordination. Stretching can even enhance your nerve impulse velocity, which refers to the exact time it often takes to transmit an impulse from your brain to your muscles than back to your central nervous system. With that, your muscle groups will start working together in a more coordinated and synergistic manner.

Lessens the Wear and Tear of Your Joints

Your joints are also among the components of your body that you must protect from wear and tear. Chronic tightness and the severe tensing of your muscles may weaken the opposing muscle groups. This can result in unnecessary wear and tear of your joints and body structures.

Stretching also helps the muscles on all sides of your joints to retain an equal level of pull. With that, your joints can move efficiently and freely in every direction. This helps not only in minimizing the stress on your body but also in promoting optimal movements.

Overall, stretching and flexibility training is important as it contributes a lot to improving the quality of your life. Despite the physiological changes you may encounter as you age, your regular stretching routines combined with range-of-motion exercises can assist you in boosting your flexibility regardless of your age. This can lead to longevity and healthier quality of life.

Chapter 4

Stretching Guidelines: Tips and Tricks in Starting a Stretching Routine

Before you start doing any stretching exercises, it is important to learn a few tips and tricks that will guide you throughout your journey, especially if you are still a beginner. Note that you should prioritize your safety before starting any fitness routine. Your safety is also something you should focus on, even if you are just planning to do simple stretches.

A crucial point to remember is that the whole stretching process should not make you feel terribly uncomfortable. It should not be forceful, too. Instead, it should be gentle. You may still feel some discomfort, but it should be mild. You should avoid forceful bouncing, too. Also, note that one of the secrets to attaining favorable results from stretching movements is relaxing while doing them.

Importance of Identifying Your Goal

Before starting a stretching routine, ensure that you have already identified your specific goals. Note that just like strengthening, you can also use stretching to achieve specific goals. Determine your goal, as this will serve as your guide in choosing the best stretching approach and exercises for you.

Your goal will also determine how often and how long you should stretch. Keep in mind that your schedule for doing this routine and the length of time you should spend for each session will change depending on what you intend to achieve.

Let's take a basic lunge or a squat as an example. Even if you see three people doing this same exercise, their individual reasons for doing it regularly will cause differences in intensity, resistance, and frequency.

This premise applies to you when you are trying to start a stretching routine. You have several reasons to stretch, and each one will require a different kind of effort and intensity. For instance, if you intend to stretch consistently to improve your performance in gymnastics, martial arts, or in your dancing or cheering squad, your stretching routines should focus on building your flexibility.

In that case, stretching should form part of your warm-up, and you must do it whenever you need to build the flexibility for the skills required in your performance.

When Should You Stretch?

Another important thing that you should be aware of before starting your stretching routines is the best time to do them. Know when you should stretch to maximize its benefits and guarantee your safety. As a guide, consider stretching your body once you feel like you have already warmed your muscles.

For instance, it could be after you warm up before your actual workout. You can also make it a part of your cool-down routine. Also, note that performing stretches after warming up and before starting a high-intensity activity may cause a sudden drop in your heart rate. That said, ensure that you elevate your heart rate again before moving on to your actual workout.

One more thing that will help you decide the perfect time for you to stretch is the fact that your muscles are usually more flexible and open toward the end of the day. This means that if your workouts are often in the evening, and you are already used to such a routine, switching it up or changing into a morning stretch will not give you a similar level of flexibility.

Recommended Frequency

It is also important to know how often you must stretch to maximize the results of this workout without harming your body. While regular stretching is good for your body, you still must avoid overdoing this activity. Many also recommend stretching for just a short period daily, instead of doing the stretches for a longer period but only a few times (probably twice or thrice) every week.

If possible, set aside five minutes for stretching every day. If you want it to be a weekly thing, focus on setting aside 20 to 30 minutes for each session. Another great piece of advice is to do it at least three times every week.

How Long Should You Stretch For?

The length of time you should stretch per session will greatly depend on your goal. If your focus is to stretch a specific muscle, holding a stretch for 30 seconds is often enough to untangle its knots. Avoid prolonging it as it may only lead to tiredness that may defeat your purpose for stretching. Stretching for over 30 seconds will not produce significant results on your muscles.

Note, though, that the 30 seconds we are talking about here are not those that you just count in your head. Use the full 30 seconds on a stopwatch or a clock as much as possible. That said, it is best to bring a timer with you when you stretch so you can really stick to the recommended length of time for stretching.

Some Tips and Tricks for Stretching Safely and Avoiding Risks

Undeniably, stretching is a great form of exercise. However, it also carries some risks if you do not do it correctly, overtrain, or overdo it.

Anyone with acute injuries should also only do stretches recommended by their doctor. In case your injury is persistent or chronic, seek the advice of a physical therapist or sports medicine professional. They are the ones who can guide you in developing a stretching plan or program that is suitable for you.

Before stretching, ensure that you have warm muscles. If you intend to stretch before your actual workout, make it a point to shake out your body prior to doing the stretch. That way, even just a bit of warmth will reach your limbs before the activity.

Also, practice vigilance. Observe your body and how it responds to the activity. The reason is that pushing yourself too hard may cause you to feel extreme discomfort and pain. If you feel that, stop immediately. If you continue, then you are only harming your body instead of benefiting it.

For you to avoid such negative effects, practice stretching safely. In that case, here are additional tips that will help you create a stretching routine and stick with it without harming your body. These tips can also help you maximize the positive effects of stretching.

Stretch as Often as Possible

You will enjoy favorable results if you stretch every day. A lot of people, nowadays, lead a somewhat sedentary or stationary lifestyle in the workplace. With that said, it is natural for the body to require a sort of warm-up after staying immobile for a long period.

Dedicating even just five to ten minutes of stretching can already provide plenty of health benefits. This duration is enough to improve your balance, flexibility, and strength. Also, note that even doing easy and slow movements in the morning will help warm your body.

Just make sure to practice gentleness when doing the movements. Avoid jarring movements as much as possible as those may only lead to muscle tear and injury. You can also enjoy better results if you hold every stretch for thirty seconds to a minute.

Warm-Up before Your Workout

While creating a daily stretching routine is important, you should also warm up your body before a workout. This ensures you don't put yourself at risk of injury during your workout.

It would be best to start slowly while taking your time instead of rushing things. This means that you should not just grab your foot right away so you can stretch your calf for just a few seconds. Doing this immediately may only put your body in danger.

Remember that any attempt to perform an exercise while your muscles are still cold or without activating or waking up your body may only hurt it. It can even further result in tendon tears and muscle pulls. To include this activity before the workout, take a short walk. You may also want to elongate your stretches to achieve the best results.

Assess Your Tension

One thing about stretching that you should constantly inculcate in your mind is that it should not cause any form of pain. So, do not forget to keep track of your muscles and how they feel every time you stretch.

Gauge the level of your tension, too. Naturally, this exercise can make you feel mild tension. However, you should avoid pushing yourself too much to the point that you have already reached that stage of discomfort.

If you begin to feel sharp sensations and pain that slowly become more severe, there is likely something wrong with your movement. Focus on just a single area if that happens. Stick to a single spot at a time to prevent pushing yourself too far. Once you start to feel comfortable as you stretch, deepen the movement without overexerting yourself.

Use Gentle Movements for Rehabilitation Purposes

Avoid pushing the end range, though. For example, the famous camel and mad cat stretch that some people perform using their knees and hands are useful for the spine's neural flossing. By moving the nerves, it is highly likely for them to develop their own space. For back pain, doing around five to six cycles of stretches before your actual training can help.

Attack Your Target Area as You Stretch

You should first scan your body to determine the specific areas where tight muscles exist. You should then attack your target spot for stretching. It should also be part of your routine to stretch your tight muscles first. Do it all the time. The reason is that these tight muscles can only hamper your ability to perform and complete the full-range workouts.

During warm-ups, utilize all your body parts' general movement as a means of scanning for tightness. After identifying them, release them by implementing the most suitable stretching techniques.

Vary Your Stretching Routines

When stretching, set the goal of working out your opposing muscles and integrating several muscle groups. This should help in building a more holistic workout. Another crucial stretching tip is changing or varying your routines frequently. That way, you will not end up getting bored.

Note that in several cases, your boredom may result in you performing your routines carelessly. It may also cause you to lose your focus. This may only make you prone to injuries. Try doing yoga workouts or participating in Pilates classes to help you find ways to vary your stretching routines and prevent boredom. Since they also focus on flexibility and mobility, these classes are excellent resources when you are trying to find new stretches.

Do Not Include Bouncing in Your Routines

Bouncing can be detrimental to your body as you stretch. If your body shifts constantly, it is highly likely for your muscles to tighten. This is not a good thing as it may only increase your risk of tearing or pulling a tendon. Try finding your focal point or balance and remain stable or steady.

If you are in doubt, use a mirror to look at yourself as you stretch. This is the key for you to determine exactly how you move, allowing you to improve your form along the process. If possible, consult a trainer or doctor to keep track of your stance and posture when stretching. That way, you can immediately correct improper forms that may cause your inability to get your desired results.

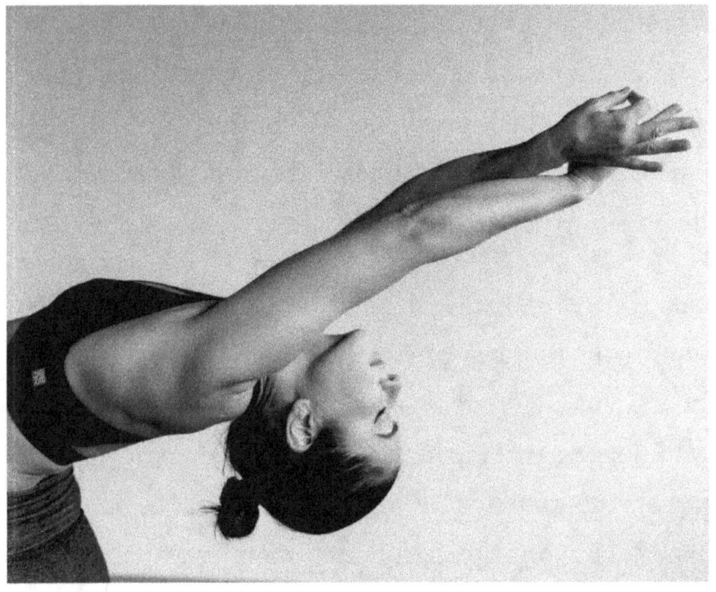

One major benefit of stretching is that it can help its proponents let go of negativities and stresses, thereby allowing them to relax their body and mind. This is the reason why you should make it a habit to breathe normally when doing your stretching sessions. Avoid holding your breath.

When deepening your stretch, allow yourself to inhale and exhale slowly. Avoid fast or abrupt breathing as it may only cause body tension. If uncontrolled, it may put you at risk of dealing with injuries. Your goal, therefore, is to make yourself feel comfortable when doing the exercise, giving your mind the chance to focus on your stretching technique.

Know Exactly Where You Should Start

With the numerous muscles composing a human body, the thought of having to stretch every day can be overwhelming. This makes it crucial to determine the specific areas you should focus on, especially if you are still a beginner. Note that you do not have to stretch all the muscles in your body at once.

If you want more mobility, the critical areas are those in your lower extremities, namely the hip flexors found in your pelvis, your hamstrings, calves, and quadriceps found in front of your thighs. You can also greatly benefit if you stretch your neck, lower back, and shoulders. Stick to a program that allows you to do daily stretches for a short amount of time or a minimum of three to four times weekly.

Also, to determine where exactly you should start with your stretching journey, you may want to seek the help of a physical therapist. This professional can help as they can make a clear assessment of your muscular strength while customizing a stretching plan or program that specifically fits your requirements.

The help of a professional is even more important if you are dealing with chronic conditions like arthritis and Parkinson's disease. In that case, it would be much better to consult your doctor first so you can start a new stretching routine that's guaranteed to be safe for you.

Learn about Proper Execution

Never stretch before getting an idea about how you can properly execute your chosen routine. In the past, most people believed that stretching was crucial for warming up the muscles and preparing them for activities. While that premise still has a bearing nowadays, it has been discovered that stretching your muscles before warming them up may hurt and damage them.

The reason is that if your muscles are cold, there is a possibility that their fibers are also unprepared, making them prone to damage. By warming up first, you can allow blood to circulate and flow to your target area. With that, your tissues will become more pliable, resulting in them being more amenable to change.

You don't have to spend a long time to warm your muscles up before you stretch. It only takes around five to ten minutes of light activities, like taking a quick walk. It is also a good idea to stretch after your weight training or aerobic workout.

To execute the stretch properly, you need to hold it for half a minute (30 seconds), at the very least. Avoid bouncing as this may only trigger injuries. Expect to feel tension while stretching, but it should not be to the point that you feel pain.

If you experience extreme pain, stop right away. It could be a sign that you are injured or there is damaged tissue. It also helps to consult your doctor and tell them about the pain you experienced so they can check the problem right away.

Chapter 5

Additional Do's and
Don'ts When Stretching

This chapter will focus on some of the do's and don'ts to keep in mind to guide you further on your journey towards achieving superior fitness, flexibility, and mobility. Remember that just like other physical activities and exercise, stretching also comes with its own rules. Try to adhere to these rules and follow them closely.

By doing that, you can increase your chance of reaching your target soundly and safely while being in good shape. So, take heed of the do's and don'ts in this chapter as they will guide you on what you should do exactly and what you should avoid when stretching.

The Do's

- **Consult a Doctor, Professional Trainer, and/or Physical Therapist** – Your safety should be your priority before starting any physical activity. Consult your doctor before starting a fitness routine that involves stretch training, especially if you have a muscle or joint injury or a chronic orthopedic condition.

It is also advisable to have a physical therapist or professional trainer assess your present range of motion and muscle strength. The assessment will be useful in creating a stretching routine that is perfect for your skills, abilities, and needs.

- **Use Static Stretching for Flexibility** – Make sure to perform this after working out, though, instead of before. Even just a few simple static stretches executed upon the end of your workout can contribute to fighting muscle soreness the next day.

- **Stretch Tight Muscles if You Train a Strong Part of Your Body** – Say, for example, you have a strong chest but tight calves. In that case, it would be beneficial to stretch your calves in between each set of your bench press routines.

To ensure that you will truly boost your flexibility through your stretches, do them often. It also contributes to increasing your stretching frequency without making the entire routine boring.

- **Use Traction Every Time You Stretch** – This is necessary for increasing your range of motion and minimizing joint compression or impingement. If you are in a gym, you can just pull on a resistance band connected to a fixed object, such as a chin-up bar or power cage.

Use your hand to hold on to the resistance band and execute a wide range of upper body stretches. Alternatively, you can perform several lower-body stretches by hooking the band onto your ankle or foot.

- **Control the Specific Area of the Muscle You Intend to Stretch** – For instance, if you plan to stretch your hamstrings, target your belly muscle every time you bend your knee, plantar-flex your ankle, point your foot away, or round your back which is crucial for optimal results.

  When locking your knee, ensure that your back remains straight. You may also dorsiflex your ankle, which means flexing your foot toward the shin. This will allow you to target the fascia, which refers to the sheath that protectively covers your muscle instead.

- **Stretch if You Think You Have Bad or Poor Posture** – Keep in mind that over time, our muscles shorten, which is a major contributor to poor posture. Your muscles may also shorten if you train consistently but with a restricted range of motion – ex. you do not execute full-range reps.

- **Target Major Body Parts That Help with Flexibility and Mobility** – These include your hips, calves, quadriceps or thighs, and hamstrings. If you want to gain upper body relief, perform stretches designed to stretch your lower back, neck, and shoulders.

- **Include Dynamic Movements in your Warm-up Exercises** – The perfect way to warm up and prepare your body for your workout is to do dynamic and low-intensity movements like the primary activity you intend to perform. Look at these scenarios.

  - **You intend to jog up to three miles** – The first thing you should do is perform dynamic movements when warming up. Walk slowly first, then speed up gradually for around five minutes. This should be enough to warm up your muscles for the actual jog.

  - **You intend to stretch your leg muscles**– In that case, perform high knee marches first. Follow them with walking lunges. Both routines can warm up your leg muscles appropriately.

  - **You plan to complete one Set of bench presses** – The first step is bench pressing using a lighter load. It should be around 50 to 70 percent lighter compared to the weight you intend to lift. Perform around 2 to 3 sets of the light presses, with 10 to 15 reps each before moving to the actual weight.

You can also perform other highly effective dynamic movements that can help you warm up, including jumping jacks, skipping rope, and arm circles. Note that low-intensity activities can slowly increase your heart rate while improving blood flow to your muscles.

These activities also work effectively in warming up the temperature of your body slowly and safely. You can, therefore, expect the activities to help you sweat out a bit, too.

- **Stretch Your Spinal Column When Performing Compressive Exercises** – Some examples of compressive exercises are overhead presses and squats. Make it a point to give your spinal column appropriate stretches in between each set.

  Note that it is not uncommon for those who follow a weight training program to lose around 20 to 40 millimeters of height. You may want to stretch your spinal column to prevent that from happening. One way to prevent spinal decompression is to hang from a chin-up bar to give the area a proper stretch.

- **Hold Every Stretch for Around 10 to 30 Seconds** – Allow your muscles to lengthen slowly and avoid forcing it. It also helps to do around 2 to 4 reps per stretch.

- **Scan Your Entire Body to See if There Are Tight Muscles** – After that, use stretching to attack the target spot. Make sure to focus on stretching your tight muscles first. Tight muscles can stop you from doing full-range movements and exercises.

It is often the case when you perform dynamic stretches prior to the actual training. When warming up, scan for muscle tightness by using the general movement of the different parts of your body. After detecting them, you can release such tightness with the help of the correct stretching strategies.

The Don'ts

- **Do Not Let Yourself Hold a Highly Intense Stretch for Over 15 Seconds** – Doing so puts you at risk of muscle hypoxia. Note that your muscles may suffer from insufficient amounts or lack of oxygen when they are under an extreme level of tension or force. This may cause more connective tissues to develop, further leading to reduced strength that will only make you inflexible.

  As much as possible, just utilize multiple angles performed for shorter durations through static stretches instead of sticking to just one angle and holding it for an extremely long period. Remember this important rule in stretching – the more intense the stretch is, the shorter its duration and application.

- **Do Not Avoid Strength Training Composed of Passive Stretches** – Make it a part of your daily fitness routines instead, as the movements here can boost your flexibility provided you do the training while applying a full range of motion. Just make sure that the movements and stretches, including the ones below, target the correct part of your body.

- o Stiff-legged deadlift for the hamstrings

- o Seated overhead triceps extension

- o Incline bench dumbbell curl for biceps

- o Flat bench dumbbell fly for pectorals

- o Seated cable row for the mid-back

- o Standing calf raises for the gastrocnemius

- o Single-arm cable lateral raise for the deltoids

- o Stability ball crunch for the abdominals

- o Lying dumbbell pullover for the latissimus dorsi

- o Seated calf raises for the soleus

- **Do Not Contract Your Muscle Right after a Stretch to Negate It** – Take this scenario as an example. When you use one hand to hold the overhead bar appropriately positioned in a power cage, then you bend your knees so you can sink down as far as possible, you will be giving your lats an excellent stretch.

The problem occurs when you also pull back with the muscles that the stretch targeted as it may only defeat your purpose. To prevent that problem, make it a point to use both your legs when coming back up from the stretch.

- **Do Not Hold Your Breath When You Perform a Stretch** – Doing so when stretching may only cause the further tensing of your muscles. What you should do, instead, is to try to relax. You can do that if you exhale longer than when you inhale.

  Remember that the opposite, which involves you hyperventilating, can excite your system even further. It may help before you perform a set of intense deadlifts, but it is not highly recommended whenever you need to stretch.

- **Do Not Let Discouragements Weigh You Down** – Avoid giving up even if your progress is slow. Remember that specific bad postures and repetitive motions take a long time to reduce mobility. A sedentary lifestyle for a long period after an injury or illness has even worse results.

  That said, avoid expecting just a few sets of stretches to bring back your complete range of movement, flexibility, and mobility immediately. It may take longer than you initially expected to restore your flexibility, especially if you are targeting specific muscles.

- **Do Not Overtrain or Overwork Your Muscles** – After attaining the perfect range of motion and flexibility for a certain joint or muscle, stop that stretching movement when you are working out. Note that if you overwork your muscles and they get excessively tired, you will only lose your progress and cause more harm than good to that area.

- **Do Not Overstretch** – This is similar to the previous tip. You must stretch then hold that muscle beyond the typical or standard length to make it more flexible. However, avoid stretching to the point that you are already experiencing pain. Dong that may only cause serious damage to your body.

You may dislocate a joint, sprain a ligament, or tear a muscle along the process. Make sure to stretch a muscle only to the point that is comfortable for you. Hold that stretch for around 15 to 30 seconds only. Avoid exceeding a minute as much as possible.

Guided by these do's and don'ts, you will be able to begin your journey towards improving your mobility and flexibility by executing safe and appropriate stretches. Probably, one of the most important tips of all is to avoid quitting. Once you start to regain some mobility and flexibility, stick with the process.

Done correctly, expect to feel and notice some progress after a few sessions. However, it would still be a lot better to have yourself evaluated by a professional trainer or healthcare professional occasionally. That way, you can accurately measure how much you have improved in terms of your range of motion, flexibility, and mobility.

Chapter 6

What Is Static Stretching and How Can You Do It?

Static stretching encompasses all stretches that you can do without movements. This form requires you to get into the appropriate stretch position then hold it for a certain amount of time. It is the most common form of stretching for beginners as it is effective and carries minimal risk and a lower chance of injury. Static stretching is perfect for beginners and those who lead a sedentary lifestyle but want to restore their flexibility and mobility.

The main objective of static stretching is to increase the length of your muscles gradually. One great thing about it is that it is suitable for everyone regardless of their age, fitness level, and weight. It is even possible for you to modify the stretches that fall under this type so they can meet the specific flexibility required by an athlete or a sports enthusiast.

The static stretch also involves stretching your muscles until you feel that there is a gentle pull. Hold it for a short period, preferably around 10 to 30 seconds only, then relax that muscle. For static stretching to work, it should be pain-free. If there is pain, it is natural for your muscles to tighten as a means of protecting themselves, so be vigilant about that.

Static stretches also work well to build your flexibility, especially after you experience a muscle strain injury. However, for strong and healthy muscles, PNF (Proprioceptive Neuromuscular Facilitation) type stretches are better for enhancing flexibility.

Advantages of Static Stretching

Incorporating static stretching into your daily routines carries several rewarding benefits, making the activity truly good for your body and overall fitness. Apart from the general benefits of stretching, it also boasts several unique positive effects.

- **Minimal Risk of Injury** – With the extensive range of motion that static stretching can provide, you can lower your risk of injury, including muscle strain.

- **Quick Recovery** – Static stretches also aim to increase the flow of blood and lactic acid absorption – both of which aid in faster muscle recovery. Quick recovery can lead to more training on your part.

- **Prevents Muscle Soreness** – Strength training may cause delayed muscle soreness, which may happen in around three days or seventy-two hours after the session. You can prevent that or at least lower your chance of dealing with that issue if you incorporate proper static stretching into your session.

- **Corrects Your Posture** – Your tight muscles tend to affect your posture negatively. Left uncorrected, they may cause significant changes in how you stand, move, or sit. You may want to do some simple static stretches to loosen those tight muscles and finally employ exceptional posture.

- **Better Performance** –Static stretches can also make your muscles more flexible, a big help in improving your performance. Regardless of what physical activity or sports you are involved in; your sports performance will surely improve with this form of stretching.

- **Improves Your Balance** – Static stretching also works to create body awareness. You can use this awareness to improve your balance. You can even expect to improve your ability to perform balance exercises – one example is a one-leg stand.

- **Fights Tension Headache** – Another unique benefit of static stretching is that it can help you relieve tension headaches. The reason is that you can also perform static stretches that target the tight muscles in the area around your upper neck. You can loosen the muscles in that area, which can lead to immediate muscle relief.

Perform regular static stretches, and you will feel a lot healthier and fitter, aside from the dramatic improvement in your overall mobility and flexibility.

Are There Downsides?

Despite the numerous benefits of static stretches, there are also instances where they can be bad for you. This is especially true if you do it incorrectly. One potential downside is that it may decrease performance instead of improving it, though this is still a rare case. This may only happen if you overdo the stretches. To be more specific, holding a static stretch for more than a minute may lead to poor performance.

Forced stretching may also happen. This may occur if you try to increase your range of motion without listening to your body and observing your limitations. You may be doing forced stretching if the activity starts causing more tightness than necessary, leading to the stiffness of your muscles.

There is also a risk that you will stretch your cold muscles. You must prevent this from happening at all costs, as forcing the stretch of your cold muscles may only injure them instead of fixing them.

To avoid the possible downsides and achieve only the best results from static stretching, you must know exactly when to execute this form of exercise. The safest times for you to do static stretches include after your strength training, after sitting in one place for too long, or driving for over an hour, and after doing an aerobic activity like bicycling, swimming, or running.

You may also want to execute a few static stretches during your training to improve your posture. Moreover, the static stretch is safe for anyone who has already consulted with a physical therapist.

This means that your consultation may have already taught you how safe static stretching is and if it can truly help reduce your pain and improve your range of motion.

Who Should Stay Away from Static Stretches?

Some people can benefit more if they do other forms of exercise instead of static stretching. If you are any of the following, you may want to avoid all kinds of static stretches as much as possible.

- **Arthritis Sufferer** – The painful and swollen joints brought on by arthritis makes static stretching bad for you. It is unnecessary as it may only worsen the health of your joints.

- **Suffers from Pain with an Unknown Source** – It would be best to visit your physical therapist or doctor before you do static stretching if you experience pain with a source, you can't identify yet. You must seek the help of a professional in determining the source of your pain, so you can determine first if the stretching exercise is indeed safe for you.

It is also advisable to avoid starting your workout or training with a static stretch, even if your main goal is to boost flexibility. If possible, let your muscles warm up and increase your body temperature first. One way to do so is to perform a quick jog. This should be enough to prepare your muscle for the static stretch.

Some Safety Tips

A static stretching routine needs to be productive, easy to implement, and fun. You can achieve all those by ensuring that you are already well-versed about some safety tips on performing static stretches – among which are the ones that we will discuss briefly next.

- **Be Gentle** – As much as possible, implement slow and smooth movements. Never do bouncing or jerking movements when trying to hold a stretch. Moreover, you should be extra cautious if you have just recovered from an injury.

- **Begin Slowly** – Make it a point to begin with only a few static stretches. You can then integrate more stretches and reps as soon as you notice your flexibility and range of motion improving.

- **Focus on Form First before Depth** – You need to do your static stretches using the right or correct form. This is the key to preventing yourself from getting harmed in the process.

For instance, you may want to check if you have squared hips or if you aligned your joints instead of forcing a deeper stretch. Note that depth will come naturally and quickly if you stretch with the right form and technique.

- **Move Smoothly as You Make Transitions** – Every static stretch movement you do has to be controlled, gentle, and slow. Stop yourself from bouncing as it may create microtears in your muscle fibers, thereby causing damage.

- **Set Your Static Stretching Session for a Minimum of Ten Minutes Daily** – This should be safe enough for you, provided you execute the stretch correctly. By stretching for a minimum of 10 minutes and doing it daily, you will notice a significant improvement in your flexibility and overall strength and balance.

When prioritizing your safety as you stretch, note that this activity may cause a little discomfort, though it should not be painful. Experiencing pain, especially after your training and exercise, is a bad sign. With that in mind, try to avoid pushing your muscles and joints past their limits.

What you should do, instead, is to develop a routine that provides you with all the benefits of static stretching without overexerting yourself. Also, always keep in mind the safety tips here and begin slowly but surely.

Easy Static Stretching Exercises for Beginners

Now that you already know most of the crucial facts about static stretching and how to safely do them, it is time to delve into the actual practice. The next section will focus on the static stretches that are simple yet beneficial enough for beginners.

Overhead Triceps Stretch

This is a static stretch that targets the muscles found in both your shoulders and around them. It stretches your triceps and the large muscles you find at the back of the upper portion of your arms. Such muscles are necessary as you use them to stabilize your shoulders and extend your elbows.

The good thing about the overhead triceps stretch is that you can use it when recovering from injury and to relieve muscle tension. Moreover, it can prevent the tightening of your muscles while boosting your circulation and keeping your connective tissues loose.

- Begin in a standing position with both your feet planted on the floor, hip-width apart. Focus on releasing tension by rolling both your shoulders in backward and downward movements first.

- Lift your right arm to the ceiling. Then bend your elbow to bring down your right palm to the middle of your back.

- Lift your left hand, then use it to pull down your right elbow gently.

- Stay in this static stretch position for 20 to 30 seconds, then switch arms.

- Perform the mentioned steps twice or thrice and on both sides. Try to get into a deeper stretch as you do each rep.

Posterior Capsule Stretch

With the posterior capsule stretch, you can target your shoulder's back when stretching. This is the perfect static stretching exercise for anyone who performs plenty of throwing or pitching.

- Start this exercise by relaxing your shoulders. Then draw one arm across your chest.

- Take the other arm and position it directly over your shoulder and hold it in place.

- Hold this position for around 30 seconds. Repeat the steps using your opposite arm.

- If possible, increase the time you spend holding the stretch as well as its depth. However, make sure that you also observe your body, and only do it to a point you can tolerate.

Hamstring Stretch

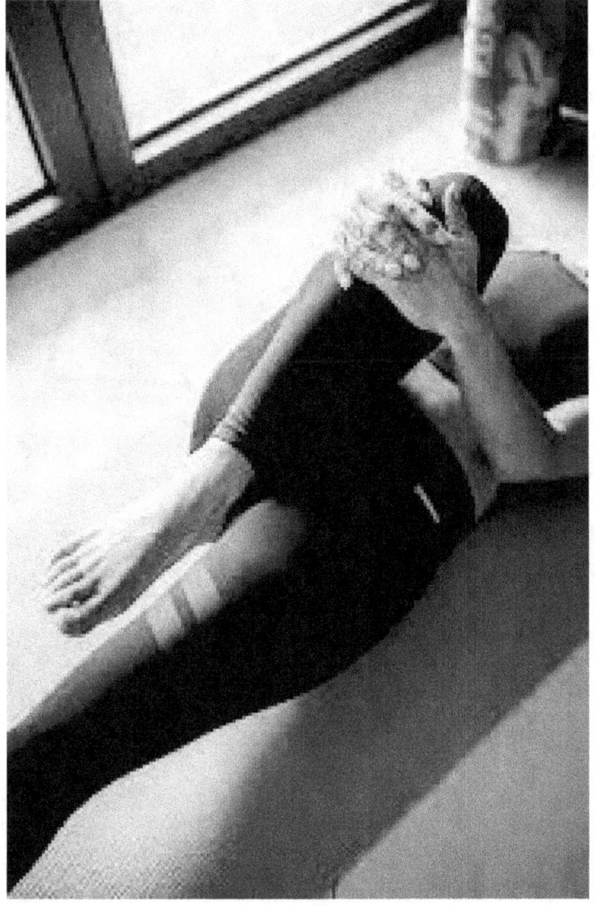

As the name suggests, this is a stretch that targets your hamstrings. It is particularly beneficial for runners. You will also find the hamstring useful if you suffer from tightness in your hamstrings brought on by sitting for long periods or having poor posture.

In addition to improving your posture and flexibility, hamstring stretch also contributes to preventing injuries and relieving back pain.

- Square your hips and place your feet facing forward.

- Place one leg on a stool in front of you. Make sure that the stool you use is low enough.

- Bend forward gently from your hips. Keep your back flat and knees straight. Continue to bend forward until you feel the stretch in the back part of your thigh.

- Hold this for a minimum of 30 seconds.

- Repeat the steps, but with the opposite leg on the stool.

Seated Butterfly Stretch

This specific static stretch targets your lower back, inner thighs, and hips. The good thing about the seated butterfly stretch is that even beginners can safely and conveniently do it. It can provide effective and immediate relief from the tightness in the hips.

This static stretch is also needed to improve your flexibility, especially after prolonged sitting, repetitive movements, and strenuous workouts. Make sure to warm up your body before performing this stretch, especially when the weather is cold.

- Sit on the floor. Make sure that your abs are tightened and that you straighten your back while you are in the seated position.

- Put the soles of your feet together while bending your knees to one side. Use both your hands to hold your feet. Draw your heels to you until you feel your hips, lower back, and thighs stretching.

- Hold this position for around 10 to 30 seconds while breathing deeply and slowly.

Biceps Stretch

The biceps stretch works on your biceps together with your shoulders and chest muscles. It is a fantastic technique that blends well with your upper body workout. The biceps stretch also works effectively in relieving muscle tension and tightness often brought on by the daily grind and stress. Moreover, it can help improve your posture, athletic performance, and strength while giving you ultimate relaxation.

- While in a standing position, place both your hands on behind your back. Interlace your fingers when your reach your spine's base.

- Straighten both your arms. After that, turn your hands with your palms facing down.

- Lift both your arms as high as possible. Do this until you notice that there is a gentle stretch on your shoulders and biceps.

- Hold this static stretch for around 30 to 40 seconds. Perform 2 to 3 reps to maximize results.

Cobra Pose

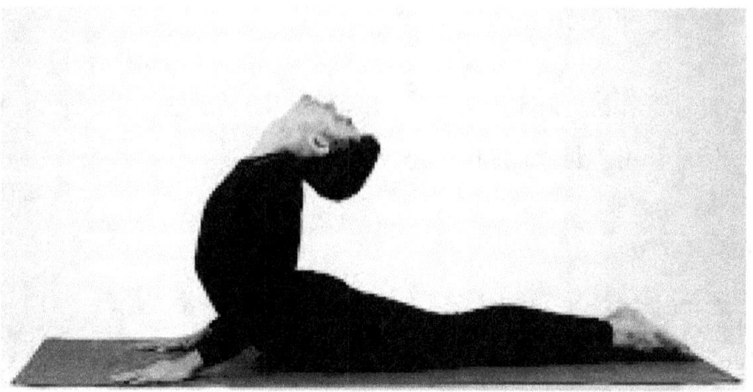

This stretch benefits your chest, shoulders, and abdominals. When performed correctly, the cobra stretch can relieve the muscle tightness in those areas.

- Lie on your stomach. Put your hands directly beneath your shoulders flat on the ground while lying on your stomach. Ensure that your fingers face forward when you are in this position and that you tightly draw both your elbows close to your chest.

- Press into your hands, keep your elbows squeezed to your torso, then lift your chest, shoulders, and head off the ground. The next step is lifting your torso partway. You may also lift it halfway or completely upwards.

- Bend your elbows a little. You may also deepen this pose while allowing your head to drop back.

- Stay in this position for 30 to 60 seconds. Do two reps.

Neck Stretch

A lot of people hold a lot of tension and stress in their shoulders and neck. If you have the same problem, then the neck stretch is the most effective static stretch that you can use for muscle release in those parts your body. You can do this pose either standing or sitting.

- While you are standing or sitting tall, put your right arm on your head's right side. Your left arm should then be placed by your side.

- Pull your head slowly to your right shoulder. Do until you feel a good stretch you on your left neck. Be gentle.

- Hold this stretch for 30 seconds before releasing.

- Repeat the steps but on your opposite side.

Stretching your glutes is vital as it can help your weaker yet tight muscles become more relaxed. Your glutes are the muscles composing your buttocks, and they are important when performing a lot of your activities, including jogging, running, cycling, and swimming. You can keep these muscles in shape with the help of this glute stretch routine.

- Start this routine in a seated pose. Your feet should be flat on the ground and both your knees should be straight.

- The next step is putting your right ankle on top of your left knee.

- Keep your muscles engaged when in this position, then press the other knee actively away from you. This is the time when you will feel the stretch in your exterior right glute.

- Hold this pose for around 20 seconds while breathing calmly.

- Repeat on the other side.

Kneeling Hip Flexor

The kneeling hip flexor is a static stretch that will loosen your hip flexors, which is beneficial as it can prevent injury. It also lowers your risk of developing hip pain. If you are dealing with back pain because of a disability or prolonged sitting, this stretch can also offer relief. Furthermore, it can correct a tilted pelvis and improve your sprinting speed.

- Begin this routine in a low-lunge pose. Bend your knees at a 90-degree angle.

- Position your leg so that your knee is directly on top of your ankle. As for the back part of your knee, align it with your hips.

- With your left hip, press forward actively while engaging your core.

- Breathe while holding this pose for around 20 seconds before moving on to the opposite side.

Head-to-Knee Forward Bend

This stretch targets many different muscles, particularly those in your groin, calves, hamstrings, and back. It also makes your lower back and spine more flexible, which is extremely important as many poses need a flexible spine and a strong back.

- Look for a comfortable surface and sit with your legs straight out in front of you.

- Put the sole of your right foot on your inner left thigh.

- Inhale, then raise both your arms overhead. The next step is exhaling while lengthening your spine then bending forward.

- Let your hands rest on the floor, your legs, or foot.

- Stay in this position for 30 to 60 seconds.

- Repeat the steps but on the other side.

All the static stretches mentioned in this chapter are truly beneficial for your body. Aside from enhancing your range of motion and flexibility, static stretching also promotes quick muscle recovery after your workouts, resulting in minimal stiffness and pain. You can also use the stretches here to release muscle tension and stress for more effective relaxation.

Chapter 7

What Is Dynamic Stretching and How Can You Do It?

Dynamic stretching consists of active movements and stretches that require your muscles and joints to undergo a full range of movement. These are safe to use when trying to warm up your body before your workout routine.

Expect dynamic stretches to be functional while mimicking the movement of the sport or activity you intend to perform. One example is when swimmers circle their arms as a way of warming up their body before finally getting into the water.

You can also look at dynamic stretches as a set of movements designed to move your body before any form of exercise. Many of those who practice dynamic stretching say that this routine can bring even average stretches to another level. Most stretch every morning as they get out of bed. Serious yoga practitioners also make it a point to spend a few months perfecting these postures.

Dynamic stretching takes these movements to a new level as it can make you feel like you are an Olympic athlete. It can also help in loosening the stiffness in your legs and arms and improving your muscle power. The only thing you have do to make this work for you is to get your body moving.

Dynamic stretching also differs from regular stretching, especially the static type, due to the movement involved in the former. For instance, you can pump a few high kicks or move your arms by circling them before your workouts to make these routines more dynamic.

Moving with these stretches gets your joints and muscles ready to work in more demanding positions. Dynamic is also different from static stretches because aside from involving movement, you do not have to hold the stretches for a specific length of time.

Who Is It For?

Among those who regularly execute dynamic stretching are professionally trained athletes. They do the stretches before they compete in various sports events. Some examples are Olympic runners and soccer players, whom you will see in constant motion as they push and strain their bodies and muscles to extreme limits.

Note, though, that dynamic stretching is not only for professionals. It also works for physical therapy patients, gym rats, and recreational hikers. Even those who are at over 65 can perform light to moderate dynamic stretches and benefit from the routines.

The intensity of your dynamic stretches often depends on your present health and age but generally, you can rest assured that they work for everyone. Low-intensity dynamic stretches that you can do for around five minutes can positively affect your muscles, especially when it comes to solving pain and stiffness.

Also, keep in mind that it is normal for you to feel some pain initially as you start your workout, but you can use dynamic stretches to ease such discomfort.

When Is It Safe to Use and Do Dynamic Stretching?

You can take advantage of dynamic stretching before starting any workout or exercise routine. It helps warm up your body and make your muscles move, thereby preparing them for the work ahead.

There are also certain scenarios wherein the dynamic stretches can produce the most favorable benefits, including:

- **Before Athletics or Sports** – You can perform dynamic stretches if you are an athlete who will either jump or run. It could be that you are a sprinter, soccer player, or basketball player. If you are any of those athletes, dynamic stretching is safe for you.

- **Before Weightlifting** – It is also safe for you to execute dynamic stretches before your weightlifting sessions as they can help in improving your performance and leg extension power.

- **Before You Do Cardio Exercises** – Whether swimming, running, or participating in a boot camp, dynamic exercises can contribute a lot in warming up your muscles and preparing them for movements. This can result in better performance while you are doing your cardio and reduce your risks of injury.

What Are the Benefits?

Like other forms of stretching, dynamic stretches also have plenty of benefits that are both similar yet unique when you compare them to the others.

Warms up Muscles for Proper Functioning

Dynamic stretches work effectively when it comes to warming up your muscles to the point that they reach the ideal working temperature. They stretch out your muscles thoroughly, which offers a significant improvement in your overall function.

Note that while static stretching effectively lengthens your muscles so they work better, it is still possible for their performance to diminish over time. Since static stretching does not involve movement, your muscles will be left cold and unprepared for a tough and demanding exercise or workout.

Meanwhile, dynamic stretching provides the advantage of getting your muscles warmed up enough that it would be easy for you to work out afterward while being less prone to injuries induced by workouts. Static stretching is effective and appropriate after a workout, while its dynamic counterpart works perfectly as a pre-workout routine.

Pumps Up Your Blood

Before working out, it is crucial to prepare not only your muscles but also your cardiovascular system. Your heart may have a harder time ramping up its beats per minute within a shorter period compared to a longer one. It is particularly true for those who have desk jobs or live a sedentary lifestyle.

With the help of these dynamic stretches, you can get your heart pumping, to get you fully prepared once you begin to work out. Aside from pumping your blood and heart, it can elevate your energy, too. The increased circulation helps transport oxygen and vital nutrients to your body quickly, which is a big help in keeping you more energized as you work out. When this happens, it would take longer for your body to tire out, giving you the chance to work out even longer and maximize its effects.

Improves Coordination

Nothing can beat dynamic stretches when it comes to their ability to help improve your coordination. Several of the stretches in this category, like the lunges with a twist and high knees, need a lot of coordination, so expect to improve in that area if you do the routines regularly. Having excellent coordination is beneficial for athletic purposes and for performing daily tasks and activities, such as driving.

Gives Good Mental Preparation for Your Workout

This is an incredible psychological benefit of dynamic stretching. It can contribute a lot to preparing you mentally for your workout. Note that aside from being physical, the whole preparation for a race, competition, or workout is also mental. No matter how prepared you are physically, you can't expect to be at the top of your game if your mind is not in it.

Dynamic stretching does not literally stretch your brain, but it can provide you with a sufficient transition time designed to help shake off all the issues in your head. It allows you to clear your head, which can help you focus on the race or workout ahead.

You can also use several dynamic stretches to reconnect with your body, giving you a chance to get a feel of what it takes to push yourself. In addition, you can use the time you spend for dynamic stretches to think of the workout goals you intend to achieve for the day.

Makes You Fully Prepared to Take on High-Intensity Workouts

In addition to warming up and loosening your muscles, dynamic stretching can also contribute a lot to performing high-intensity workouts. The fact that you will be relaxing your muscles and increasing your range of motion from this exercise is enough to prepare you for a highly intense exercise.

It can give you sustained power, muscle endurance, agility, strength, and anaerobic capacity. Moreover, it can lessen muscle stiffness, thereby preventing you from experiencing discomfort, soreness, and stiffness when performing HIIT. Dynamic stretches are also highly recommended before performing high-intensity exercises as they prepare your joints for the activity, which can eventually prevent injuries.

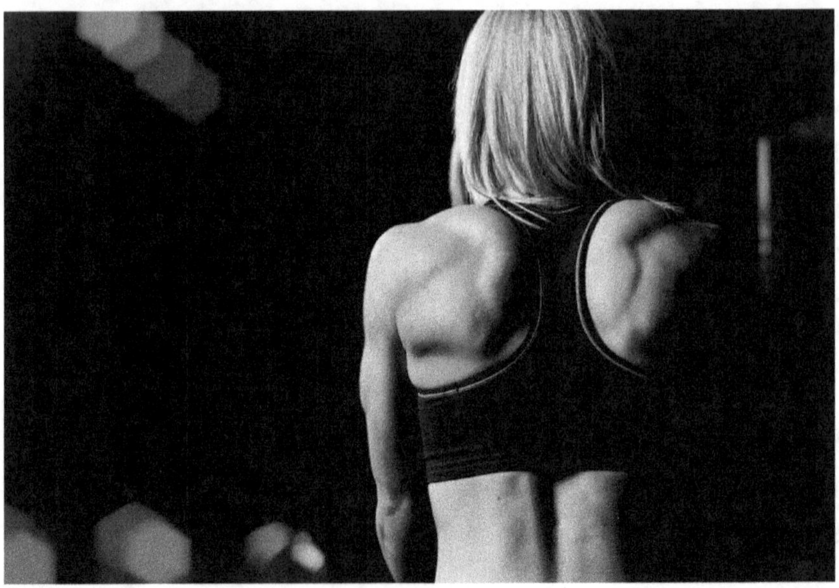

The enhanced muscle power brought on by regularly doing dynamic stretches is also a huge help in making you run longer or taking on more weights. Dynamic stretching is also a much better choice than static if your goal is to improve your ability to lengthen your workout. Attaining a more extensive range of motion is also another benefit of dynamic stretching that is vital for you if you wish to engage in physical activities for a longer period.

Getting Started with Your Dynamic Stretching Routines

The first thing you should do to begin a dynamic stretching routine is to pick a workout or sport you intend to focus on. This step should also involve choosing the kind of stretching you should do. For instance, you may want to mix static and dynamic stretches together to make them even better for your body.

After learning about the stretches you wish to try, select the primary muscle groups you want to target first. In most cases, the muscles prioritized by a lot of practitioners are the bigger ones, including the quadriceps, glutes, and hamstrings.

You should then determine how much time you will commit to your chosen dynamic stretching exercise. If possible, aim to get around ten to fifteen minutes of dynamic stretching prior to every training session to maximize the benefits of your workout.

Safety Tips

- **Begin with Basic Dynamic Stretches** – Avoid moving to complex stretches right away, especially if you are still a beginner and have no stretching experience. Just start with the simple and basic moves, then transition into more complex ones based on your agility and comfort level.

- **Use an Assist** – Do not hesitate to use an assist if you are still new to the concept of dynamic stretching. It could be a pole, wall, or weight bench that you can hold onto when doing the stretch.

You can use anything that will help make the dynamic stretches and movements easier to do. Once you become more used to the routines, you can finally let go of the stabilizers and begin relying on the innate strength of your body.

- **Consult Your Doctor if You Have an Existing or Acute Injury** – Perform only those stretches that your doctor recommends. In case of physical limitations that cause difficulties in doing a stretching exercise, you should also talk to your doctor first to determine the best alternative exercises designed to boost your flexibility.

- **Avoid Dynamic Stretches if You Are Older than 65** – It would be much safer for seniors to do static stretches instead.

- **Be Careful Not to Overstretch** – Note that one of the biggest downsides of dynamic stretching is that it makes you prone to overstretching. That said, you should be mindful of the capabilities and limitations of your body.

Listen to what your body tells you whenever you do the stretches to lower your risk of injuring yourself when warming up. If you are not careful, you will end up dealing with the negative side effects of overstretching, including muscle strains, swelling, ligament tears, and bruising.

- **Begin with Slow Movements, Then Slowly Increase the Intensity** – That way, your joints can naturally adapt to the movements and attain maximum mobility.

Top Dynamic Stretches to Try

Now, it's time to start learning about the specific dynamic stretches that you can do. The dynamic stretching exercises compiled in this section are among the best that can significantly help improve your training and workout sessions.

Arm Circles

The arm circle is an effective dynamic stretching routine used frequently by runners. Make sure that your arms are widely extended to maximize the effects of this move on your joints. The arm circles also work in building the endurance of your shoulders while lowering your risk of suffering from rotator cuff injury.

Note that because your shoulders have an extended range of motion, it is important to warm them up thoroughly and arm circles can help with this.

- Begin by standing with your feet shoulder-width apart and parallel to each other.

- Extend both your arms to the sides, parallel to the floor, then perform wide circular movements with both your arms.

- Increase the speed through which you execute the circular movements but make sure to do it gradually.

- Do 10 reps forward and 10 reps backward.

- Finish 2 to 3 sets of arm circles to maximize its results.

Spinal Rotation

This dynamic stretch targets your upper body, which is an excellent warm-up before you lift weights. Your spine is made for supple movements, but with the modern and sedentary lifestyle that most people practice nowadays, it has also become a source of non-movement.

You can refresh your spine using this spinal rotation exercise to restore your connection to your body. It can also help your spine regain flexibility while easing your neck tension, opening and relaxing your chest, and removing tension from your jaw.

- Lie down on your back. Make sure that you bend your legs with your feet flat on the floor, and you keep your arm outstretched while in this position. Alternatively, you may bend both your arms at the elbow in case you lack space.

- Breathe in then out. While breathing out, twist your legs bringing your right knee, followed by the left slowly to the floor.

- Hold the pose for only 5 to 10 seconds, then return to your starting position.

- Repeat the steps but do them on the other side.

If you feel good about doing this stretch, you may also choose to rotate your head in the legs' opposite direction. Stick to slow and controlled movements all the time.

Lunge with a Twist

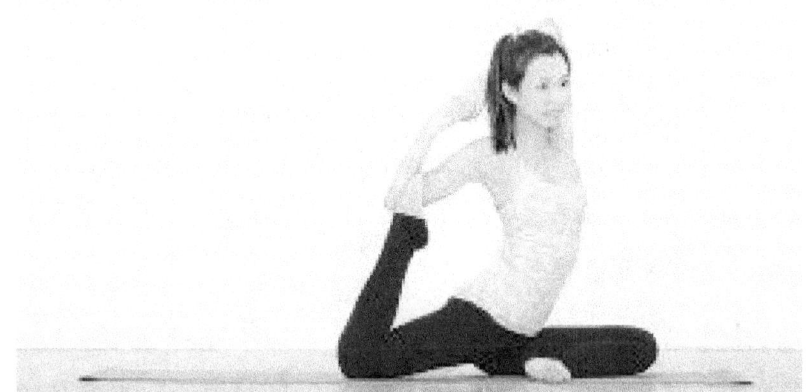

The lunge with a twist offers the remarkable advantage of engaging your core, glutes, and legs. You can also isolate the hamstrings and quads in your legs as you perform the lunge. You may want to add a twisting motion to this routine, and you can choose to do so along with added weight.

By doing that, you can contract your glutes more fully while engaging your core. This dynamic stretch is also what you need to keep the muscles used in performing exercises engaged. This is especially effective for activities that require the use of one leg after the other, like running, cycling, and cross-country skiing. The lunge with a twist can also form part of rehabilitation therapy for those who just went through hip surgery.

- Stand tall and upright with your feet are planted on the floor, shoulder-width apart.

- Use your right foot to step forward. Lower your body into the basic lunge position. Avoid letting your right knee go beyond your toes.

- Starting from your midsection, twist your upper body to the right. Engage your core while doing so. Also, make it a point to squeeze your glutes while taking extra caution to avoid rotating your knees.

- Let your torso go back to the middle using slow and controlled movements.

- Finally, put your right foot back to return to your starting position.

Leg Pendulum

The leg pendulum is also a worthwhile addition to your dynamic stretching routine because of the many benefits it can provide. For one, it can strengthen your balance and endurance. It also boosts and extends your circulation. All these benefits are what many sports and fitness enthusiasts and athletes need in general.

- Start by swinging one of your legs back and forth. The other leg should remain balanced when you are doing this activity. If necessary, hold onto a wall for proper support and balance.

- Swing your leg forward and backward 5 to 10 times.

- Put it down, then do the swinging again with the other leg. Repeat it 5 to 10 times.

- You may then swing both your legs from one side to another while facing the wall if you want.

Dynamic Arm Swings

The arm swings are highly effective dynamic stretches capable of engaging your upper body muscles. Aside from warming up and stretching your arms, shoulders, upper back, and chest, the dynamic arm swings also help prepare your joints, tendons, and muscles for your workout. It can also provide an immediate cardio and flexibility boost. Doing the dynamic arm swings regularly can loosen up your torso and arms.

- While facing forward, extend your arms in front of you. They should be at the height of your shoulders with your palms facing down.

- Walk forward while swinging your two arms to the right. Your left arm should reach the front part of your chest, while the right arm should extend out to your side.

- While swinging your arms, retain the position of your torso, which means that it should continue facing straight. Turn only the joints on your shoulders.

- Reverse the swing's direction to the opposing side while walking.

- Repeat the steps 5 times per side.

Walking Lunge

The walking lunge is one of the best dynamic stretching exercises you can do if your goal is to target your glutes, hip flexor, and hamstring. Doing it regularly can help in attaining unilateral leg function and strength. It can also boost leg hypertrophy while establishing a connection between real-world function/movement and strength training.

- Stand upright with your hands placed on your waist.

- Step forward, then perform the lunge.

- Align your front knee with your ankle and hip, then lower the knee of your back leg to the floor without letting it touch it.

- Make sure that your front knee does not go past your toes as you execute the lunge.

- Push the back of your leg, then use your opposite leg to step forward, allowing you to lunge in a similar fashion.

- Make use of the muscles in your abdomen and prevent your back from arching.

High Kicks

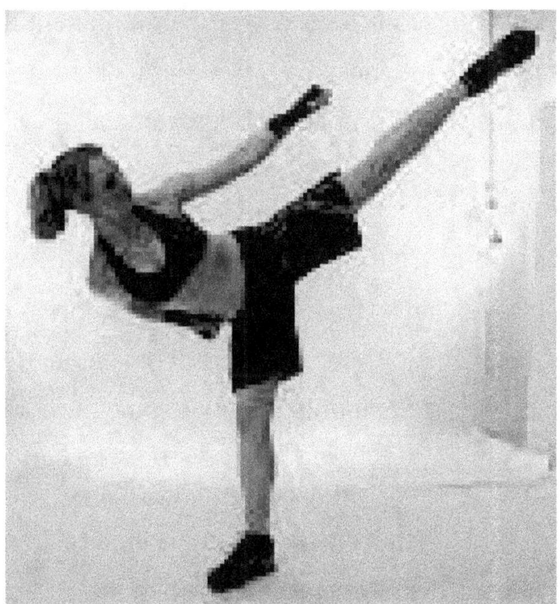

This dynamic stretch is an excellent warm-up routine that targets your glutes and legs. It is beneficial for anyone who executes it as it can significantly strengthen the core and lower body while making the hamstrings more flexible. A wise tip is to speed up your movements, as doing so will help pump up your heart and burn calories.

- Straighten your left arm out in front of you.

- Stay in that position while kicking your right leg high up in the air. It should be as high as the palm you have just extended.

- Perform five kicks before switching sides.

One important tip when performing the high kicks is that if you are incapable of touching your foot to your palm, make it a point to let yourself go as high as possible. Be extra cautious, though, to prevent your hamstrings from being overextended.

Trunk Rotation

The trunk rotation is what you need if you want to warm up your whole body through an extensive range of motion. You will find this exercise helpful in improving your core strength, flexibility, and stability. It also works in making your spine more mobile.

One more advantage of trunk rotation is that you can do it in various ways. With that, you have a high chance of progressing, challenging yourself, and performing variations of trunk rotation movements that you know are suitable for you.

- Begin this exercise in a supine position. This means lying on your back. Bend your knees and ensure that your feet remain flat on the floor.

- Position your upper body and shoulders in a way that you can maintain them firmly against your exercise mat or the floor.

- Extend or outstretch your arms, then have them pressed to the floor. This should help in attaining balance as you execute each move. Tighten or engage your abdominal muscles during this step.

- Rotate your knees slowly toward the ground to one side. Do this while still sticking with your range of motion and with controlled movements. Expect your feet to shift but ensure that they stay on the floor.

- Hold this pose for around 3 to 5 seconds.

- Tighten or engage your abdominal muscles so you will have an easier time moving your legs to the other side. Hold this pose for 3 to 5 seconds more.

- Remain focused while practicing normal breathing throughout the whole exercise.

- Do the exercise again for a certain number of reps – for instance, 10 reps per side.

Scorpion Stretch

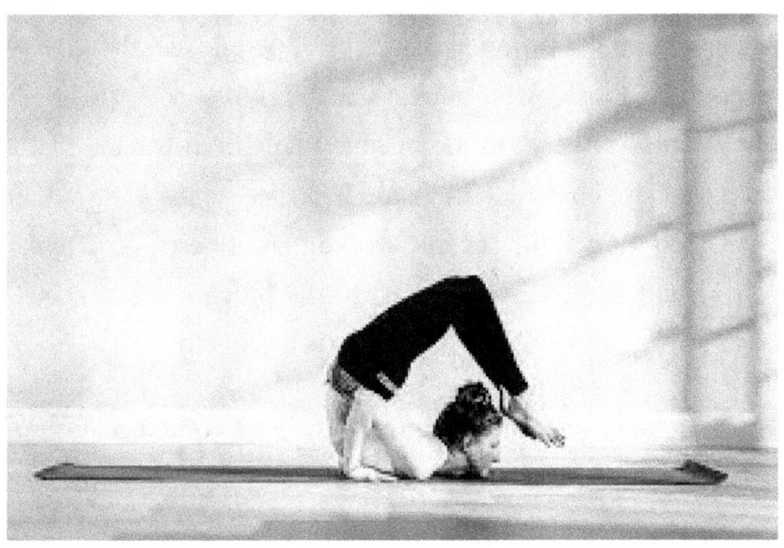

With the scorpion stretch, you can take advantage of the ultimate solution move for your mobility and flexibility issues, especially one brought on by sitting for too long. You should consider performing this dynamic stretch because it does not target just one muscle, rather, it targets several muscle groups while promoting hip mobility. Among the muscles that the scorpion stretch works on are the glutes, quadriceps, hip flexors, and the muscles in your shoulders and chest.

- Lie down flat on the floor face down and stretch your arms out to the side to form a "T" with your body.

- Next, roll your body to your right, while keeping your arms outstretched and bring your left heel across your body.

- Do the same step for the other side.

Squats

Squats are a common routine that a lot of people are already aware of, especially those who exercise regularly. What's great about squats is that they serve as a dynamic whole-body stretch that also works as an effective warm-up routine. The squat is so common that you can find it in several workout routines. As a dynamic stretch, it will surely give your body the preparation it needs for your workout session.

- Start in a standing position with both your feet positioned hip-width apart.

- Lower your body slowly and gently so you can get into a squat position. Ensure that both your knees do not go beyond your toes.

- Squeeze your glutes, specifically the muscles in your buttocks, when you go back to your initial standing position.

- Repeat this move 10 times.

With all these dynamic stretches, you will no longer run out of movements that will help in warming up your body. Again, just be extra cautious if you are injured. Try limiting your physical activities in that case. Stop anytime you feel like the stretch or move triggers some sort of pain.

Also, remember that some dynamic stretches may only strain your body and are unsuitable for those with specific health issues. For instance, the squat may just add more stress to your joints if you are suffering from arthritis or knee injuries, so it would be best to stay away from them. It is also vital to maintain proper form and slowly and safely execute your movements rather than injure yourself.

Chapter 8

The Difference between Passive and Active Stretching

Active and passive stretching are two methods used by athletes to work actively towards improving their mobility. Both are sub-categories or sub-types of static stretches, but it is crucial to delve deeper about the two for you to get to understand them, especially how they work individually.

Both active and passive stretching can also benefit you in various circumstances, and the use of each one frequently depends on the specific situation you find yourself in. If you want to work out frequently but find yourself constantly sitting hunched over your phone or computer, you should integrate a mobility and flexibility routine into your weekly workouts.

Active Stretching Defined

As one of the methods used in enhancing one's flexibility, active stretching is all about actively contracting one muscle to stretch its opposing muscle. You can do this without any external force. This method is also called static active stretching, which means that it is non-moving. It requires you to hold the stretch's end position for a certain amount of time.

What makes active stretching distinctive is that instead of seeking the help of a prop, like a band or a strap, you hold your stretch simply by using other muscles. Generally, the hold will be for 10 to 15 seconds. It is important to try not to go beyond that period, otherwise, you may experience difficulties along the process.

An example of this is when you lie on your back while you are on the floor and lift your leg straight up to the ceiling. You can do that until you feel and notice the stretch in your hamstring. To hold such a position without using a strap requires your core and hip flexors to work actively to ensure that your leg stays up in the air. On the other hand, your hamstrings or the muscles positioned opposite your hip joint stretch statistically.

Passive Stretching Defined

Meanwhile, passive stretching refers to a form of stretching exercise that requires the use of an external force. This means that you will need the help of a person or an object to stretch instead of doing the stretching actively. You can often accomplish this stretching method by performing partner stretches, using stretching accessories, or gravity so you can gain assistance.

Any stretching routine that depends on an external force can be considered passive. In addition to being effective in improving your flexibility, passive stretches are also worthwhile to include in your cool-down routines. This makes them different from active dynamic stretches that you can use as a warm-up and effectively promote the flow of blood to the target muscle groups before an activity.

What Are the Clear Differences?

Speaking of differences, let's delve deeper into the different areas that make passive and active stretches different from each other.

Execution Time

The first area that makes passive and stretches different from each other is the timing. For active stretching, you need to do it before the start of your workout. It tends to serve as a warming exercise capable of flexing your muscles before you do an intense workout.

Passive stretching is one that you can do after your workout or exercise. Some even consider it as a post-workout or cool-down exercise. You can do it to give your muscles sufficient time to relax after going through an intense workout session.

Exercise Routine Execution

You will also notice a few differences in the way you execute the individual routines. For the active stretch, you will most likely do it by standing straight in just one position. You should never dwindle as you raise one leg slowly in front and allow it to remain there for around 10 to 15 seconds. You can repeat the steps 4 to 5 times.

It is also possible for you to modulate the routine. You can do so if you lift one of your legs then raise it backward. Ensure that both your hands are parallel to your shoulders. Meanwhile, your head must be lifted while looking straight. It is a big help in retaining balance. Complete a rep by sticking in that position for 15 seconds.

As for passive stretching, the usual routine involves you holding the legs of an active participant while you are doing the exercise. The active participant must lie on their back while facing the ceiling. While your partner is in that position, stretch your legs. This should be enough to exercise or work out your hamstrings.

Another way to do the passive stretch is to let yourself lean against a door then slowly lift one leg. Hold that position for around 10 seconds. Repeat it using the other leg. You are also allowed to use the floor and let yourself lie down. Ensure that your chest is against the floor as you do it.

Lift yourself from that position so that you can exercise your arms. You may also want to stretch your legs next to the floor to promote a more revitalizing exercise under the passive stretching category.

Required Equipment

The two methods of stretching also differ based on the equipment required when executing them. Most active stretches, for instance, do not require the use of any equipment at all. What you must use is the strength of the opposing muscle.

Meanwhile, passive stretching requires the use of equipment. It may come in the form of support, like a floor, a machine, or a wall. You may also do the passive stretch with the aid of someone, like a partner, as you perform your exercise.

Offered Benefits

There are also a couple of differences in some of the benefits that active and passive stretches offer. For instance, active stretching can benefit your opposing muscles, also called the agonist, by making them flexible. It is also the recommended stretching method for runners as it can help in strengthening their agonist muscles.

It is also advisable to carry out the active stretch daily, specifically before you workout or start your running session. The reason is that it aids in boosting your athletic performance while lowering your risk of suffering from an injury.

On the other hand, passive stretching is more beneficial for those who aim not only to increase their flexibility but also improve their endurance. However, when you indulge in a passive stretching routine, keep in mind that incorrectly doing it may only affect you adversely.

It may only lead to you suffering from excessive pain and injury. Your ligaments are prone to stretching and tearing if you execute positions incorrectly.

Active Stretching Examples

Now that you know how the two differ, it is time to learn a few active stretches that you can do regardless of whether you are at home or work. Before that, it is important to learn a few guidelines that will help you execute them correctly.

- Pick a muscle you wish to target when stretching, then choose a corresponding move or pose.

- Flex the opposing or agonist muscle.

- Stay in that position for 10 seconds or so or until you notice some stretching sensations in the muscle you targeted.

- If you intend to do a bilateral stretch, one involving your arms and legs, you can just repeat the steps again for your other limb.

Active Hamstring Stretch

The first active stretch that we are going to talk about is the active hamstring stretch. As suggested by its name, the active hamstring stretch indeed targets your hamstring. This stretch aims to improve your strength while enhancing your flexibility.

Such an exercise also works in reducing muscle fatigue and injury as well as promoting blood circulation. In addition, you can increase your stamina and improve your balance with the help of this active stretching routine.

- Begin by lying on your back. If necessary, put a pillow below your head as it helps produce good blood flow. Straighten your two legs on the floor.

- Raise one of your legs to the ceiling while making sure that it consistently remains straight. Do this until there is already a stretch in the area. Once you feel the stretch in your hamstring, hold the position for around 10 to 50 seconds.

- Observe your tailbone. If it starts to tuck in, slightly lower your raised leg. You may also bend your leg at the bottom and gain the support needed for this exercise by putting your foot on the floor.

Active Glute Stretch

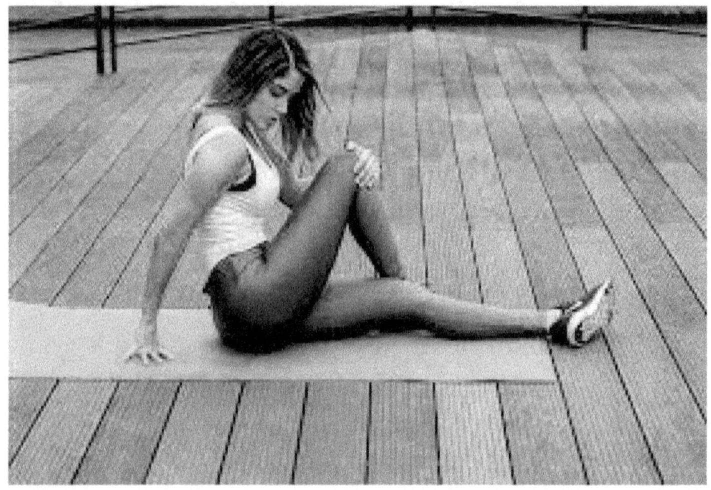

As the name suggests, this specific active stretch targets your glutes – a group of muscles composing your butt. Note that this should not cause you any pain, so avoid pushing yourself too hard in case you suddenly feel some pain and discomfort.

- Sit on the floor while putting both your legs straight out in front of you.

- Prepare to bend your right knee. After that, bring it over the opposite thigh (left).

- The next step is to position your right foot in such a way that it lays flat on the floor.

- Your left elbow should then be placed outside your right thigh.

- Twist the upper part of your body gently to the right, then hold this pose for around 10 to 15 seconds.

- Repeat the steps on the other side.

Active Triceps Stretch

Your triceps are also among the most important muscles of your body that can be improved with the help of an active stretch. Your triceps are the muscles located at the back of your upper arm, from your shoulders down to your elbows.

- Stand straight. Make sure that you practice good posture when doing so. Point one arm straight up to the ceiling without lifting your shoulder.

- Bend your elbow. Do this while you move your hand down behind your neck. Make your hand reach in between your shoulder blades.

- When doing this stretch, your goal should be to continue pointing your elbow to the ceiling. Let your hand reach down your back even further. This pose should take around 10 to 15 seconds.

Active Chest Stretch

This type of active stretch mainly targets your pectorals or chest muscles. When performed correctly, this active chest stretch can also give your biceps the stretch they need for more flexibility.

- Begin in a standing position. Maintain good posture while standing straight.

- Using both your arms, reach out to your sides at a 90-degree angle. Ensure that you have straight elbows when doing so. This can help in increasing the stretch once you turn your palms either toward the ceiling or forward.

- Open your arms wide. They should be opened wide enough that you can extend them behind your body. Stop once the stretch is already felt across the front part of your arms and your chest.

- Stay in that pose for 10 to 15 seconds. Ensure that your ribcage does not flare and your back does not arch from this stretch.

Active Quad Stretch

The quads refer to the group of muscles located at the front of your thighs. This is what you are going to target when doing the quad stretch. To make this activity easier to do, you may want to put one of your hands either on the wall or a chair so you can maintain your balance.

- Stand tall. While standing, position your feet hip-width apart. Maintain not only a good posture but also a neutral pelvis when in this initial position. If you want, put one of your hands on a chair or wall for proper balance.

- Bend one of your knees. Lift the foot behind you, then aim to touch your butt. Continue pointing down your knee to the floor. It also must be in line with the knee supporting it.

- Hold for 10 to 15 seconds.

One more reminder when doing the active quad stretch is that flexing your hip or putting your knee forward may only reduce the stretch, so be extra cautious.

Passive Stretching Examples

You should never forget when performing passive stretching exercises that you must do them after working out or doing a warm-up sufficiently. That way, your muscles are already warm, resulting in more relaxed muscle fibers that lead to a more beneficial and deeper stretch.

Another guideline is to hold a stretch that falls under the passive category until you notice a release in the targeted joint or muscle. Some of the stretches here require a partner. In those instances, you must clearly communicate to your partner whenever you feel like you have had enough of the stretch.

Also, note that some passive stretches may take longer due to the required time to hold a specific pose. Despite that, committing to doing the stretches is worth it as you can see positive results quickly.,

Lying Knee to Chest

This passive stretching exercise requires you to follow a recovery position. It is a great technique if you plan to stretch out the front part of your legs while also releasing your hips. It is an incredible stretch that you can do at any time to help you relieve stress. Just make sure to look for a comfortable place where you can lie down when doing this exercise.

- To start, lie on your back. Straighten both your legs in front of you.

- Pull up one knee to a 90-degree angle toward your chest. Ensure that your shin face the ceiling.

- Wrap your arms around your knee. You should then pull it to your chest.

- Continue pressing the other leg directly against the ground. This should help in creating resistance and the required stretch targeting your hip.

- Let your back and hip flexors relax while in this recovery pose.

- Hold for a minute, then do the steps again on the opposite side.

Seated Side Bend

You may want to do this passive stretching exercise if you have noticeable tightness in your hip flexors and sides. The good thing about the seated side bend is that you can do it regardless of your level of flexibility. The only thing you need is sufficient space where you can conveniently extend your legs.

- Start with a sitting position. Extend your right leg straight to the side. As for your left leg, bend it towards your right knee.

- You should then stretch or lift your left arm atop your head.

- Next, slide your right arm along your right leg toward your toes.

- Stretch your left arm over your head and bend your torse toward your right foot. Wait for the stretch in your left side.

- Let gravity do its job of pulling you naturally closer to that leg. Provide some space for the left part of your body.

- Hold this pose for around thirty seconds, then do it again on the other side.

- Repeat the stretch on the two sides once more after you have completed the set.

Forward Fold

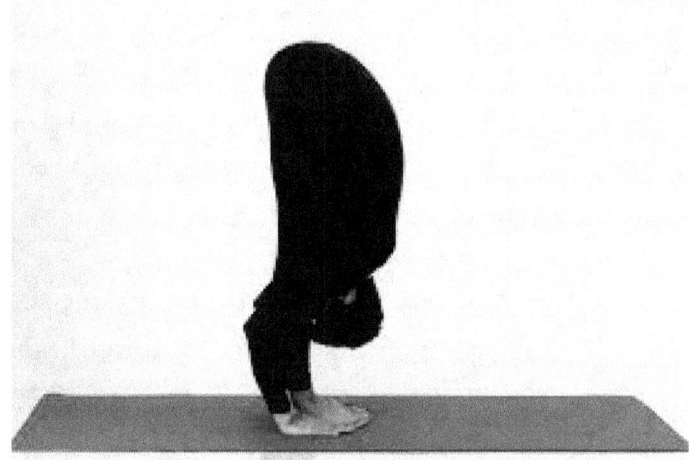

The forward fold is a great passive stretching exercise that you can do regardless of your current flexibility level. It particularly helps those with tight hamstrings since gravity will be of help in this stretching routine. It does not require any fancy equipment either. If you want to maximize the results of the forward fold, it is advisable to repeat it thrice daily. This should be enough in lengthening your muscles.

- Start the forward fold by standing straight up with both your arms positioned by your sides.

- Your chin should then be tucked on your chest. After that, roll down to the floor.

- Use your arms to reach the floor. This should also be the time when you let your head's weight drop naturally.

- Stop every time you feel like there is a mild and gentle stretch. Continue the routine while you allow gravity to pull you down naturally.

- Hold this stretch until you feel the release of your hamstrings.

Piriformis Stretch

Also known as the figure-4 stretch, you can execute the piriformis stretch if you plan to target your piriformis and glutes. It can also improve the flexibility and mobility of your hip muscles while relieving tightness in the area.

- Lie on your back. Bend your right knee and lift your left leg and place your left ankle to cross over your right knee.

- While in this position, grab your right thigh. After that, pull the right thigh to your chest. Make sure that your left knee points directly to the side.

- Hold this position for around 20 to 30 seconds. Do the same steps again with the other leg

Supine Single Leg Stretch

This specific passive stretching routine can provide your body with several benefits – one of which is the increased flexibility that it can give your hip flexors. It also gives your legs and back a proper stretch while strengthening your core. Moreover, it flexes your upper body during the entire session, which is a big help in boosting your endurance and stamina.

- While lying on your back, lift your left leg. Make sure that you continue keeping this lying position straight.

- Prepare your right leg so you can fully extend it straight out. Alternatively, you can bend your knee, so you can put your foot down, planted on the floor.

- Interlace your hands as you put them behind your left calf or thigh. Get a strap or towel, then put it around the bottom part of your foot.

- The next step is to pull the left leg toward your body using your hands, a strap, or a towel. Do this as you also press back your leg gently. This should help in resisting movement.

- Hold this pose for a max of one minute while retaining normal breathing.

- After that, you can finally release your leg, but do so slowly and safely. Continue doing the stretch by going over the steps on the other side as well.

Standing Quadriceps Stretch

The standing quadriceps stretch allows you to stretch your quads as a means of boosting the flexibility of this huge muscle found in the front part of your thighs. You can often see this stretch as part of the after-exercise stretching or the warm-up routines of many people, especially those whose activities include running, yoga, and cycling. While you have various choices when it comes to stretching your quads, this version is quick and simple and you can do it while standing.

- Stand on your left leg, placing your left hand on a wall or chair to help you balance.

- Bend your right knee and bring your heel to your buttocks.

- Place a towel or a strap around your ankle (the right one, specifically), or use your right hand.

- Pull your foot gently to your body while pressing a foot against your chosen resistance.

- Hold the pose for a max of one minute while maintaining normal breathing patterns.

- Release the right leg slowly, then repeat the procedure while focusing on your left leg.

Reclined Butterfly Stretch

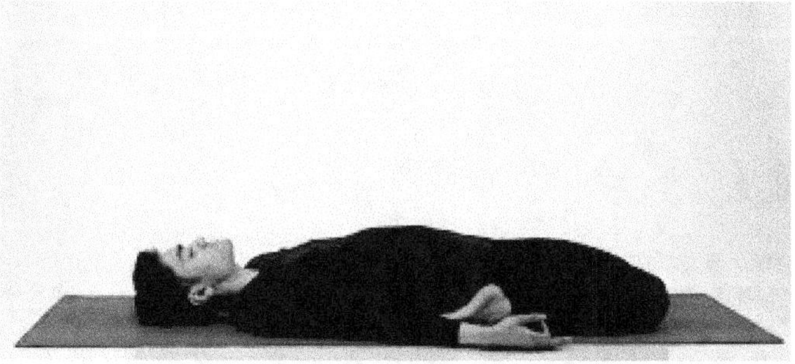

This passive stretching exercise is one that you can do with the help of a partner. The reclined butterfly stretch also carries several advantages – one is that it can make your inner thigh adductor muscles, the muscles used in drawing both legs together, more flexible.

You can expect this stretch to help retain your balance and stability while opening your hips, which may become tight due to prolonged sitting. What's even better about the reclined butterfly stretch is that it is safe to do even for pregnant women.

- The first step is to lie with your back on the floor. Press your soles into each other. Your knees should also be positioned in a way that they are open to the sides.

- Let your partner put pressure gently on the lower part of your thighs. While your partner does that, push both legs against such kind of resistance for around ten to thirty seconds.

- Do 1 to 3 reps and allow yourself to relax between each set between 5 – 10 seconds.

Chapter 9

Ballistic Stretching and How to Do It

Ballistic stretching is a stretching method that requires you to use a body part or limb's momentum so you can force it, albeit briefly, to go past the range of motion that's normal for it. It is different from static stretching, which requires controlled and slow motion, gradually pushing your body to the natural range of motions.

In ballistic stretching, you will have to go beyond such limits, challenging your body differently. The two stretching approaches are different, but they can also complement each other based on your chosen routines. Just like static stretches, the stretching exercises under ballistic also have their unique set of positive and negative qualities.

Ballistic stretching is also different from dynamic stretching. Both stretching methods may require the use of movement as you stretch, but they are completely different. One difference is the fact that dynamic stretching does not require pushing your muscles beyond their natural range of motion. It does not also involve any momentum or bouncing.

Doctors, therapists, and fitness experts recommend static and dynamic stretching rather than ballistic for beginners. However, it still pays to understand what this form of stretching is, so once you get into the stage where are ready to do it, you already have an idea of what it is all about.

Who Is It For?

As you may know by now, ballistic stretching can be defined as a warm-up stretching technique involving sudden and quick movements designed to boost flexibility. Athletes and those who exercise every day are the ones who use this form of stretching mainly to increase not only their range of motion but also muscle power.

You can do it by using momentum and bouncing so you can execute a hyperextended stretch. Ballistic stretching also seems to fit the requirements of dancers, basketball players, martial artists, ballerinas, and other sports enthusiasts and athletes looking for a safe way to stretch in order to boost their jump momentum and flexibility.

It is also advisable to perform ballistic stretches only when suggested by a coach and under the guidance of an expert for safety purposes. It can greatly benefit athletes who need an advanced range of motion to excel in the field that they are in.

Also, take note that not all sports and athletic activities require a high level of ROM. A higher level of flexibility can even reduce an athlete's strength and power output, eventually leading to decreased performance in some cases. With that in mind, it is a requirement to seek the advice of experts first, whether your present activity or sports requires you to execute ballistic stretching every day to excel.

Unique Benefits of Ballistic Stretching

Performed by the right set of people, ballistic stretching is beneficial as it provides a lot of rewarding benefits.

- **Challenges Athletes** – One remarkable advantage of ballistic stretching is that it continuously challenges athletes in a way that they will be motivated to improve their skills and abilities gradually while setting new records. The whole exercise involves pushing your body beyond what is comfortable or normal for it. It is, therefore, perfect for physically intensive activities.

- **Provides a Dramatic Increase in Flexibility** – Of course, improved flexibility is a common benefit among all types of stretching routines, but the kind of flexibility that you can get in ballistic stretching will help improve your performance in whatever sports or physically intensive activity you preform. Note that sports like volleyball, basketball, gymnastics, soccer, martial arts, and even dancing require superior flexibility.

  With ballistic stretching, you can push your muscles through their limits. A pre-workout session composed of ballistic stretches can, therefore, help train your muscles and prepare them for high-impact activities. This kind of stretching can even significantly increase vertical jumping, which is great for basketball players.

- **Lower Risk of Injuring Your Tendons** – In comparison to static stretching, ballistic stretching is more effective in preventing the possibility of tendon injuries. It can also significantly lower the stiffness in your Achilles tendon. Moreover, it can help prevent muscle soreness.

- **Better Muscle Motor Performance** – To achieve this positive effect, it is advisable to perform a warm-up routine for around 5 to 10 minutes before engaging in a ballistic stretch. If you are an athlete, then the regular execution of ballistic stretches can minimize your muscle soreness, which can significantly boost your athletic performance.

Eventually, it can help in toning your muscles and joints, allowing them to work and fire faster using more power and force. With this specific benefit, it is no longer surprising to see a lot of athletes viewing ballistic stretching as the most effective technique for warming up.

- **Better Blood Circulation** – With the ability of ballistic stretches to warm up your body through a set of rigorous and demanding exercises, expect an increase in your blood flow that every part of your body will experience.

This increase in blood flow also increases the possibility of your body receiving more oxygen, which in turn helps to heal your tissues faster. To enjoy this benefit, though, several athletes and trainers recommend doing static stretches first before moving into ballistic stretching.

- **Elevates Your Energy** – You will also be amazed by the ability of ballistic stretching at getting rid of any lethargic feelings. If you feel groggy or tired the entire day, you can use ballistic stretches as a means of alerting you while charging your body with a higher level of energy.

Furthermore, these high-intensity workouts result in higher calorie burn, which can contribute to weight control. This is beneficial, as excessive weight gain can cause you to feel exhausted and lethargic most of the time.

Possible Risks and Dangers

Despite the many benefits of ballistic stretching, you should still remember that it is often designed for more experienced practitioners. It is meant for those who are already used to high-impact and high-intensity activities, like athletes involved in sports that really test the capabilities of their bodies. It also works for those who are already used to working out every day.

If you are a beginner, you may want to train using other forms of stretches first before trying ballistic. It will also do you a lot of good if you consult your doctor or therapist first and find out if ballistic stretching is something you can do.

Some of the risks that you will most likely face when doing ballistic stretches are:

- **Sudden and Forceful Stretching Movements That May Hurt Your Ligaments and Soft Body Tissues** –Overly forceful movements can cause damage to the soft tissues surrounding your joints, including your tendons and ligaments. This may eventually lead to tendonitis. Small muscle tears will form over time that can only reduce your movement and flexibility.

- **A Higher Level of Susceptibility to Injuries for Your Muscles and Tissues** – The rapid bouncing action that you may have to do leads to a higher risk of injury. The sudden jerky movements may stretch your joints and muscles past their capacity, which is good for those already used to it but not so much for beginners. It can also result in excessive muscle tension and the potential of a muscle tear.

- **Prone to Being Performed Incorrectly** – Since ballistic stretches force your body to go beyond its typical limits, many experts still warn those who try these exercises not to overlook the possibility of injuries. The problem is that ballistic stretches are prone to be executed improperly and incorrectly, raising the risk of injury. One example is when you do the ballistic stretches too quickly or too hard.

It doesn't matter if you are new to this form of stretching or an athlete who is already used to high-impact activities. It is still a must to perform the ballistic stretches with regulated movement and aptitude to guarantee your safety. Doing it with the assistance of an expert is also important.

Some Safety Tips and Precautions When Doing Ballistic Stretches

Before you can reap all the benefits offered by ballistic stretching, you must be one hundred percent sure that it is indeed the most suitable kind of stretch for you. Also, ensure that you properly learn each movement and correctly execute it.

Remember that if you poorly and incorrectly execute it, you will only be putting your body at risk. That said, never do ballistic stretches unless you are already well-equipped with the most helpful safety tips and precautions during the execution.

- **Consider Some Vital Factors** – Among them are your present body shape, size, and age. Consider your physical condition as well before you practice ballistic stretching. For instance, an adult who is out of shape may be prone to injuries if they do ballistic stretching suddenly and without proper guidance.

  If you are a beginner at physical activities, you should also consider the amount and level of stretching you can safely do. Think about your overall physique and fitness, especially if you suffer from a joint, ligament, or muscle-related condition or injury. If you are a professional athlete, find out first whether ballistic stretching is the most appropriate stretching method for you.

- **Warm Up Adequately** – To perform ballistic stretches safely, you must make sure that your body and muscles are already in motion. You can make that possible by warming up before engaging in ballistic activity first. In that case, you may want to do a few cardio exercises.

  If possible, set aside around 5 to 10 minutes to warm up your body. This should help increase your body's internal temperature, making it more supple to the point that it can handle stretching even further.

- **Seek Professional Guidance** – Since ballistic stretches come with their own risks, make it a point to hire a professional and expert trainer who can guide and assist you throughout the stretching process. This can assure you that you will be doing the whole ballistic stretching process without pushing yourself too much and too far. This will also prevent you from unsafely and incorrectly executing motions.

  If you are still uncomfortable incorporating ballistic stretches into your workout routine, integrating a combination of static and dynamic stretches would be a safer alternative.

- **Determine the Most Appropriate Reps (Bounces) and Time per Session** – Both of these will depend on whether you intend to perform the ballistic stretch for a competition or use it as a separate routine designed to boost your flexibility.

If you plan to use it as part of the preparation for your performance, the average time for ballistic stretching is around three to five minutes while you flow from one stretch to another. Also, stick to doing around 5 to 10 reps per stretch, but this will still vary based on how you feel as an athlete. In most cases, athletes may execute a stretch but don't take it all the way if they start to feel any discomfort, then try to go back to it later after sufficiently warming up their body.

If your goal for doing a ballistic stretching routine is to turn it into a separate session to enhance your range of motion, consider increasing the time you spend doing the ballistic stretch. You may also want to look for stretches that are similar to the typical routines.

Every stretch also must contain several sets composed of a max of 20 reps. This will differ based on how well you perform as an athlete as well as your specific requirements.

- **Choose Sports-Specific Stretches** – It can also do you a lot of good if you perform ballistic stretches that involve the muscles that you mostly use in your physical activity or sports. For example, if you are into soccer, it would be more beneficial for you to stretch your hamstrings. The reason is that the sport you regularly engage in makes you more prone to experiencing hamstring strains. So, going for ballistic stretches designed to help your hamstrings will help you enhance your performance and minimize muscle strains.

Ballistic Stretching Exercises

Now, let's focus on the part where you will learn a few ballistic exercises you can try. Keep the safety tips and precautions mentioned a while ago in mind. Also, remember that just like other forms of exercise or any time you add a new stimulus, it would be best to begin with a low intensity routine.

Since you will be doing ballistic stretches, the entire process means that you must keep the bounces small. It also means practicing them with minimal force. Once you notice your body becoming more accustomed and familiar with the stress, start increasing the force and size that you use.

Make sure to control the force, though. Avoid using all your force and power while doing the exercises here to prevent getting injured. Again, you should have the help of a professional personal trainer.

Standing Lunge

This is a common ballistic exercise that you can incorporate into your other stretching workouts. It can greatly benefit your body's glutes and quadriceps.

- Keep one foot forward while leaving your arms freely hanging on both sides of your body. You may also keep your hands completely straightened out over your shoulders.

- Bend your foot forward, then quickly plummet forward. Bend the other foot behind.

- When doing this exercise, aim to put your body weight on your foot's heel as you bend it forward.

- Once you complete this routine with one foot, return to the original position. Repeat the steps but use the opposite leg.

Straight Leg Kicks

This ballistic stretch targets your hamstrings and core. It helps in loosening up your hamstrings while engaging your core. The straight leg kicks also helps your hamstrings be prepared for explosive action, like when you need to jump while serving. It can also lower your risk of suffering from an injury while boosting your hamstrings' flexibility by keeping your muscle tissue temperature high enough.

It is highly recommended to do this ballistic stretch in a more controlled manner, especially if you have not perform any warm-up exercise beforehand. The reason is that it may pull on hamstrings that are still cold. Having flexibility issues in your hamstrings may also prevent you from kicking your leg up to the level of your hip without having to flex your knee.

- Make sure to keep your leg straight while facing forward.

- Lift that leg as far as you can in front of you.

- Make the opposite or ipsilateral hand touch the toes of the leg you have lifted.

- Release your leg by putting it back down to the ground.

- Repeat the above-mentioned steps on the other leg.

Alternating Side Lunge

The alternating side lunge aims to open your hips while engaging the many major muscles that you can find in your legs. It can target your quads, glutes, inner thighs, and hamstrings. It also works in strengthening your outer thighs, calves, and core. The alternating side lunge also has the advantage of improving your agility and dynamic balance while enhancing your athletic performance and overall flexibility.

- Stand tall and straight while ensuring that your feet remain hip-width apart.

- Use your left leg to step out to one side. With your left knee bent, push your hips back.

- Go back to the initial position, then repeat the steps using the right leg.

- Continue alternating your legs until you have completed your desired number of sets.

Standing Toe Stretch

Standing toe stretch helps in stretching your hamstrings. It can target the muscles in your abdomen by mixing the crunch and the toe touches. It can also stretch the muscle groups that are present at the back of your thigh.

The standing toe stretch can even give your erector spinal muscles, the ones in your lower back, the kind of workout they specifically need. When done correctly, it can also improve your shoulders, calves, abdominals, and butt.

- Stand upright.

- Begin bouncing, then jerk down to touch your toes.

- Do it repeatedly, preferably up to 10 times though you still must consider your comfort level. Try to exceed your usual range of movement with each rep.

Hip Flexor Max Motion Range

This is another ballistic stretch that can provide a couple of benefits. For one, it helps in strengthening your leg muscles and your hips. This stretch also works well for athletes in the short or long jump.

- Stand upright with both your feet are shoulder-width apart. Shift your weight onto your right leg only so you can shift to the right part of your body.

- Begin stretching your left leg and ensure that your hip is out when doing so. As for the left leg, ensure that it is in a straight position. Only your foot's heel should be touching the floor. Your toes should be pointing directly upwards.

- Remain still for around 10 seconds. Do this movement again by using the left side of your leg. By this time, you will notice your flexors becoming more active and your hips stretched out.

Torso Stretch

The torso stretch can help in maintaining strong torso and hamstring muscles. The entire routine works in gently massaging one side of your hip while your torso turns to the other side to boost blood circulation. It can also help in flexing your muscles.

- Stand with your feet wider than the distance of your shoulders, stand upright.

- Start turning your torso side to side. You can do that if you touch your right leg using your left hand and vice versa. Do this while ensuring that your back remains in a straight position.

- Breath out each time you switch sides. Do the whole exercise for around five minutes, then repeat the steps 15 times.

- Avoid shaking your body. Keep standing still while performing the motion.

Shoulder Rotations

This specific stretching exercise works effectively for baseball pitchers. It helps them in improving the flexibility of their chest muscles.

- Begin this exercise by standing in an upright posture.

- Extend your arms to your sides and straighten them.

- Make sure that your palms are facing the room while your elbows are a bit flexed.

- Flex your shoulders as a means of moving your arms behind multiple times.

The mentioned stretches that fall under the ballistic stretching category are indeed favorable for a lot of athletes. Just don't forget that they also carry the risk of damage and injury. There's always a risk that you will pull or strain a muscle if you are not careful.

Exercise caution whenever you need to do ballistic stretches that are too forceful, otherwise, you will risk damaging the soft tissues surrounding your joints, like your tendons and ligaments. You should not do ballistic stretches unless an expert has recommended them to you.

Chapter 10

What Is Isometric Stretching?

Isometric stretching is another technique that works even for beginners. Many also consider it as a type of passive stretching. This means that it does not need any motion. For isometric stretching to work, you need tension or muscle group resistance using isometric contractions.

Static or isometric contraction also happens when you create tension in a particular muscle group without changing its length. You can use a wall, chair, the floor, or someone to serve as your resistance as you work on getting an isometric stretch and static contraction.

By far, isometric stretching provides the easiest method of developing static-passive flexibility. Some also find it more effective than doing an active or passive stretch alone. One fact about isometric stretching you should remember is that it is demanding on the joints, tendons, and muscles. That said, you should avoid stretching a specific group of muscles more than once daily.

How Does Isometric Stretching Work?

Once you contract a muscle, expect some fibers to contract while others will stay at rest. It works in the same way as when some muscle fibers lengthen while others remain at rest every time you stretch a muscle. As you perform an isometric contraction, some fibers that are resting and not involved in the stretch will most likely be pulled upon by the contracting muscles from both ends. This can result in the stretching of some resting fibers.

When there is an isometric contraction, you can't expect the number of fibers stretching to be extremely high or significant. You can only say that there is a true and effective isometric contraction taking place when a muscle, which is in a stretch already, gets subjected to such a contraction.

If you hold it long enough, several muscle fibers already stretched prior to the contraction can overcome the stretch reflex. This can eventually cause a lengthening reaction, which will inhibit the contraction of the stretch fibers. This further results in a higher level of flexibility, one that goes beyond what a passive stretch typically provides.

The use of an isometric approach on your target muscles will also cause some resting fibers to contract. However, many of them will also stretch. The lengthening reaction prevents most of these stretched fibers from contracting, which is why they stretch even more.

When you have a relaxed isometric contraction while the contracting fibers already go back to their typical resting length, expect the fibers that were stretched to maintain their capacity to stretch beyond what they can normally handle. This is a sign of flexibility.

One reason why it works is that there is a signal that tells that muscle to contract voluntarily. It also signals the muscle spindle fibers that it is the right time to shorten. This can result in the increased sensitivity of your stretch reflex, the one that will dictate your muscle spindle reaction as your muscle shortens when you contract. Your muscle spindles will also become more familiar or accustomed to the lengthened pose.

Who Is It For?

One fact about isometric stretching is that it carries the risk of harming your connective tissues and tendons. That said, it is not ideal for those with growing bones, particularly children and adolescents.

You should also avoid using isometric stretches in targeting an injured muscle, though there are instances when they can be of help as you go through the process of physical therapy. This is especially true if you are still in that stage where you need to rebuild the strength surrounding a joint or muscle that was injured previously.

In addition to boosting your ROM (range of motion), isometric stretching also aims to build your strength while you are in a stretched position. This is a good thing as the lack of strength while you are in a stretched position is a huge concern as it may trigger injury.

For instance, if you have weak hip abductors and attempt to figure out how far you can reach when doing a straddle split, you will most likely get to a point where your legs will start sliding further apart. This simply means that you are not strong enough to handle that stretched position.

The Benefits

Isometric stretching also has a huge set of benefits, provided it is carried out and practiced by the right people.

- **Activates Muscles** – One huge benefit of isometric stretching is that it promotes muscle activation, which takes place when your muscles recruit motor units. The higher number of motor units recruited, the stronger and better muscles you will have. With the help of isometric stretches, you can recruit more motor units. This can lead to stronger muscles capable of working a lot harder.

- **Supports the Rehabilitation of Joints and Muscles** – Your muscles require healing after going through surgery or anything that injures them as well as your joints. Note, though, that the entire healing process does not necessarily mean you just have to let your muscles rest without doing anything. You can work them out a bit through isometric stretches.

What's great about these routines is that they can slowly rehabilitate your joints and muscles without excessively straining them. This makes them great for those who are still recovering from previous joint problems.

The main reason is it is not a requirement in isometric stretches to move your joints. They can, therefore, keep your muscles strong without risking your joints.

- **Increases the Size and Strength of Your Muscles** – It can result in strong muscles because it increases the tension in that area while you perform the isometric stretch. By tensing your muscles for a specified period, a wide range of compounds and chemicals can stay within them, causing their growth. Doing regular isometric stretches can give you up to a 5% increase in the strength of your muscles every week.

- **Helps with Building Your Endurance** – It is also possible for isometric stretching to build your endurance, which may happen because of the constant tension applied to your muscles. Aside from that, isometric stretches work effectively in engaging all motor units. This increases the capacity designed to retain your strength and eventually surge up the level of your endurance.

- **Improves Your Posture** – Executing isometric stretches promotes ease in practicing good postural habits. It has a static nature that will help train your muscles to work effectively in building good posture because of the lack of movement. It uses muscle memory during the training so you can hold a good posture for a long period.

- **Low Impact** – Another thing that makes isometric stretching so good is that it is a low-impact routine. It allows you to enjoy its positive benefits without excessively straining you. The fact that it is a low-impact stretching routine also means that it is safe and friendly for beginners.

Are There Downsides?

Isometric stretching also has its own set of risks and downsides – among them are mentioned below:

- **Slows Down the Response of Your Muscles** – It could be due to the static contraction that may only reduce the speed through which your muscles respond. If performed incorrectly, it can slow down your performance.

- **Not That Exciting** – Some find the isometric stretches boring. One reason behind this is that most of the stretches here require you to press against someone or something static. You must do a few sets of it, too, making the whole process dull and lacking in action.

How to Do the Isometric Stretch?

To execute an isometric, stretch correctly, you need to know the general steps that most practitioners follow.

- Begin with a passive stretch that prioritizes the muscle you are targeting.

- Contract the target muscle isometrically using a static or non-moving object. Do it for 10 to 15 minutes.

- Complete the routine by letting the target muscle relax for a minimum of 20 seconds.

Some trainers also suggest that you can safely hold the isometric contraction for more than 15 to 20 seconds. However, it is unnecessary. The maximum time you can do the isometric stretch and enjoy its benefits is 20 seconds. It is also advisable to keep your stretches at max efficiency, specifically time versus results, to ensure that the stretch will not consume too much of your time.

Additional Safety Tips

Ensure that you are also safe when doing the isometric stretch. Luckily, there are a lot of safety tips and precautions that you can now access if you have plans to do the isometric exercise or stretch.

Squeeze Hard

Note that this exercise requires you not to depend on movement as a means of causing fatigue to your muscles. In most cases, it is necessary to squeeze them hard. Technically, it is called maximum voluntary contraction. It means that you can tighten your muscles based when you want to.

Breathe Properly and Correctly

An isometric stretching routine may cause you to tense up completely, which will eventually lead to you holding your breath. The problem is that when you do that, it will only cut off the thing that's needed in enhancing your performance, which is oxygen.

What you should do, instead, is to breathe properly. With eyes closed, just put your right palm on the lower part of your belly. Inhale while you visualize yourself filling up a balloon. This could make your belly rounder.

When inhaling, try pushing air out via your nostrils. Observe the way your low belly contracts. Continue inhaling and exhaling for up to five counts so you can familiarize yourself with the process. Here, you will notice your hand falling and rising together with your breathing. It is how you can breathe when doing the isometric.

Retain Correct Form

Remember the importance of maintaining proper form all the time as an incorrect and poor form may only result in injury. For instance, if you have poor form and force yourself to bench press a hundred pounds, such an extra weight can damage your lower back or shoulders.

Aside from the mentioned tips, it is also crucial to adhere to these general guidelines and tips.

- Ensure that you leave around 48 hours between each stretching routine.

- Do only a single exercise for every muscle group per session.

- Complete two to five sets of your preferred stretching exercise for every muscle group.

- Hold at least one stretch for around ten to fifteen seconds in every set.

- Those who are below 18 should not perform an isometric stretching routine.

- If you decide to make it a part of a workout or exercise session, warming up for around 5 to 10 minutes by doing dynamic stretches and light aerobic exercise can help.

- Avoid doing isometric stretching if it is not recommended to form part of your warm-up. You should also avoid doing it on the morning of the competition. The reason is that this stretch is too intense, causing it to impact your power performance. With that said, it would be much better to do dynamic stretches instead.

Isometric Stretching Exercises

With your knowledge about isometric exercises, you can finally start doing a few stretching exercises that fall under the category. The good news is that you can choose from a wide range of isometric stretching exercises available right now. Your choice should always depend on the specific muscle group you are targeting.

Split Squat Hold

This is an isometric lunge stretch that works effectively in stretching your hip flexors. It works out your quads and activates your glutes, too. Moreover, doing it regularly can significantly improve not only your balance but also your core strength.

It is a fantastic way of increasing your range of motion, especially if you experience challenges and difficulties going deeper into your lunges:

- Step with one foot forward so you can be in a wide lunge position. With your chest kept tall and nice, retain the balance on your back foot's ball as well as your front foot.

- Your back knee should then be dropped to the ground. As for your front knee, you must bend it at almost 90 degrees while sinking down as low as possible in the lunge position. Meanwhile, your back knee should just hover over the ground.

- Ensure that your front heel stays down while you keep on centering your weight and holding the bottom of your split squat.

- Continue standing tall and with a wide stance of your chest. Squeeze the glute of your back leg as a means of extending your hip. The lower part of your back should not arch, too. That way, your torso will keep on holding its nice and tall stance.

High Plank

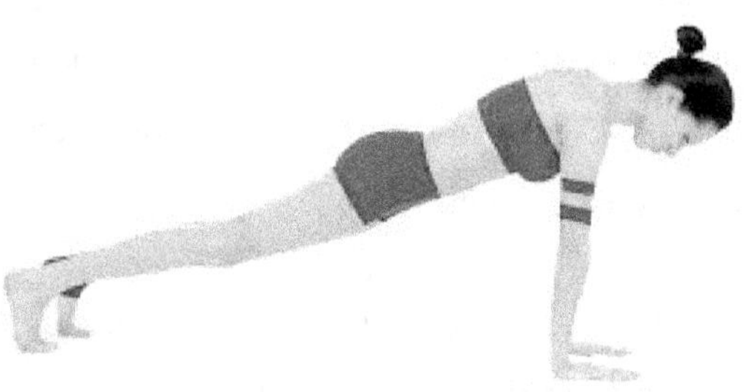

As one of the most practiced forms of isometric stretch, the plank has a lot of variations. One of these involves holding your body and resting on your forearms for a long period. It is a favorite among those who perform isometric stretches regularly as it can strengthen the core. It also offers benefits to the quadriceps, abdominals, as well as the shoulder's anterior part. For this specific variation, here are the steps.

- Start by setting yourself up into a push-up position. Ensure that your spine is positioned in a straight line.

- Press down on the floor, pushing your body away from it. This pose should result in the broadening or extension across your chest.

- Keep engaging your core while practicing deep breathing.

- Remember not to lift your butt too high nor drop your hips too low while you are in this position.

Scissor Hamstring Stretch

Another highly effective and beneficial isometric stretch is the scissor hamstring stretch. It targets your legs and gives them proper movements as it stretches both your hamstrings and calves, which can significantly improve the mobility of your hips and ankles. It also needs plenty of stability as a means of retaining balance while holding the pose.

Note, though, that for beginners, the scissor hamstring stretch is kind of challenging. If you are a beginner, it would be much better for you to use a yoga block or a wall where you can place your hands on. The reason is you may have a hard time reaching the ground.

- Step with one foot forward to get into a wide split stance. Drive down your back foot's heel while letting your front foot remain flat on the ground.

- Continue to straighten both your legs, then bend over to place both hands on the ground. The next step involves pushing back your butt while hinging over.

- Breathe while relaxing into a stretch. Sink deeper into the stretch while relaxing.

- Keep your legs straightened out even if it involves putting up your hands on something else, like a wall or the yoga block, rather than on the ground.

Low Squat

You can also take advantage of the low squat if you are looking for the most effective isometric stretching exercise. The low squat is a good exercise as it can provide your back and hips with better leverage. It can also strengthen your posterior chain, plus it is a feasible stretching technique for those who have compromised mobility.

- Stand tall while maintaining the hip- to shoulder-width space between your feet. Put both hands on the sides while pointing your toes forward.

- Maintain a position wherein you brace your core while your back remains flat. The next step to do is push back your hips.

- Bend both knees, then extend both arms forward. Lower your body depending on how far it can handle.

- Hold this pose for a certain amount of time.

When performing this isometric stretching routine, one mistake you should avoid is the inability to sit back far enough. You can resolve this by preventing both knees from going beyond your toes.

Glute Bridge

The glute bridge is also another isometric exercise that carries plenty of rewarding benefits for your body. It may be a quite complex isometric routine, but it can keep your glute muscles, core, hips, and lower back engaged. It also works in the building and strengthening of your butt, eliminating pain in some parts of your body, and improving your entire performance.

- Lie on your back. Place your hands on the floor next to your sides while lying down.

- Push your lower back to the ground, then push it up. This step should help in tightening your glutes.

- Hold the pose for around 20 to 30 seconds. After that, you can go back to your initial position.

- Do around 10 reps to maximize its effects on your body.

Twisting Half Moon

This technique works by stretching the outer parts of your hip and your calves, hamstrings, groin, and glutes. It is a great addition to your workout routine as it helps improve your balance and the strength of your leg and core, as well as your hip mobility. Note that this pose requires twisting, which makes it a fantastic solution if your goal is stretching your back and alleviating or totally preventing low back pain.

- Start this exercise with a standing split stance. While in that position, rotate to your standing leg. Keep your opposite hand down on the ground while reaching the hand that's aligned with the standing leg to the ceiling.

- Rotate your chest to the standing leg. Open it up to the ceiling. Remember that it is okay if the hip in line with the raised leg drops a bit. This can help you feel that there is a stretch out of your standing leg's hip.

- Breathe, then rotate more to your standing leg while keeping it straight. If you have problems rotating and making your hand stay on the ground, prepare a block or a stack of books where you can put your hand in.

Planche Lean

This specific isometric stretching routine also carries a few benefits. One of these benefits is that it can promote locked arm strength. The good thing about being able to maintain solid lock arms is that it will let you master several power moves, including the back lever, human flag, and planche.

- Start by getting yourself into a plank position. Ensure that you have locked elbows when you are in that stance. You also must stack your shoulders vertically above your wrists.

- Rotate wrists to around 45 degrees, then turn over your feet in such a way that you rest atop the foot.

- Your shoulder blades should then be protracted across your back. Pull these shoulder blades down, thereby ensuring that they remain depressed.

- Once all the mentioned steps are already in place, start leaning forward. Aim to make your shoulders be in a forward position, specifically in front of both hands. Avoid picking your hips. Your goal should be shifting the bulk of your workout to the upper part of your body.

Forearm Plank

Forearm plank refers to an isometric stretching exercise, providing you with the ultimate support for all your activities. The reason is that it mainly focuses on strengthening and stabilizing your spine while targeting your core muscles.

Note that the core muscles tend to contract isometrically. You can expect the forearm plank to mimic such kind of contraction, making it possible for your core muscles to begin working towards stabilizing your spine.

- Start by positioning your body in a forearm plank.

- Maintain a straight line for your spine while keeping your abs tight as much as possible.

- In several cases, those who practice it try holding this pose. However, you can also choose to contract your abs so you can benefit your core even further.

Also, take note of this tip when performing this stretch – rather than allowing your butt to hike too high or fall, focus on keeping your shoulders, knees, ankles, and hips in line with each other.

Bent-Over Press

The bent-over press is effective in working out the muscles in your shoulders and chest. Make the most out of this stretching exercise by relaxing all the tension in your face, such as in your jaw and brow. Breathe during the entire exercise, too.

- Start by positioning your body in a low lunge.

- Put both hands in a wall. They should be around the same level as your chest.

- Lean to the wall, then push. Bend down as far as you can. This should help you target your shoulders even more.

- Hold the pose for 20 seconds. After that, you can pause a bit then do 4 more reps.

Bridge

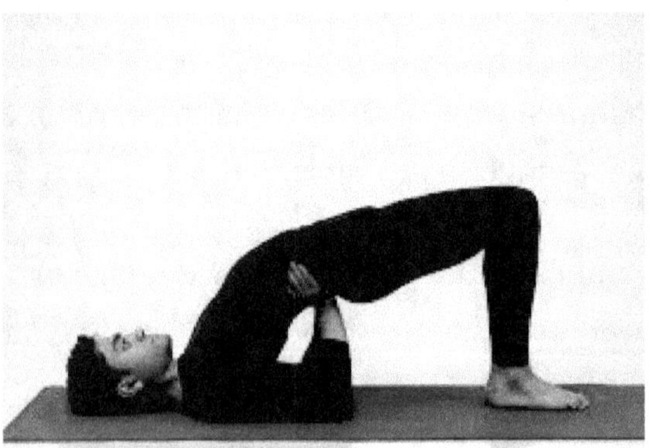

The bridge is also another famous isometric exercise that supports the goal of anyone who practices it to improve their flexibility, mobility, and strength. This specific exercise works in improving your overall strength and posture while easing lower back pain. Some of the muscles targeted by the bridge as you perform it regularly are the obliques, rectus abdominis, glutes, and erector spinae.

- Begin this routine by lying down with your back planted on the floor.

- Bend both knees while ensuring that both your hands are only on your sides. Your palms and feet should also remain flat on the ground.

- Get the support for your body from your feet and palms while you thrust your hip gently upward.

- Hold the bridge pose for around 10 seconds before you lower your body and return to your initial position.

All the isometric stretching exercises tackled in this chapter can give you all the benefits that they promise, provided you do them correctly. It is also advisable to stick to the standard period through which you should hold the isometric stretch, which is up to 30-60 seconds only. The same max length of time should stand regardless of switching positions, like when you must change to a different leg.

Chapter 11

Stretching for Seniors

Regardless of your age, you must maintain a high level of flexibility and mobility. Flexibility is always a vital part of your overall fitness and health. It is even more important for seniors. This does not necessarily mean that you should be able to split or turn yourself into a human pretzel even if you are already in your senior years. What you should focus on achieving, instead, is the flexibility to move without or with only the least restrictions.

You will enjoy your senior years even more if you can move every joint and muscle fluidly. It also promotes ease in performing your daily activities. You can do them without restrictions and the pain and discomfort that stiff joints and tight muscles may bring.

One thing to note about stretching for seniors is that you must do everything cautiously. You need to know the exact requirements for regaining flexibility without putting yourself in danger. Note that any form of exercise may be risky for seniors, especially if you consider that some body functions also decline as you age.

Despite that, with proper caution and the recommendation of your doctor and trainer, you can do various forms of stretches that are safe for you. Also, take note that executing the recommended stretches for seniors occasionally can't provide you with your desired results. You must do them regularly as suggested safe by your doctor.

You also need to be informed about a wide range of factors that can affect your result – among which are the length of time to hold stretches, how frequent you should do it, correct ways to do it, and what you should avoid guaranteeing your safety. You also must remember that stretching for seniors requires consistent effort and patience.

Length of Time to Hold the Stretch

If you intend to do dynamic stretches, perform each stretch for only a few seconds per rep. Also, be observant about how you respond to know if you are already feeling the stretch. Target around 8 to 12 reps per area with a stretch that you must hold for around 30 to 60 seconds.

Make sure that you also stick to a period that will not overwhelm you too much. By sticking with a period for stretching that is not too overwhelming for you, there is a high likelihood that you will commit to the routine and achieve your desired results along the process.

Use your body as your guide when determining if you already have enough of the stretch. Observe what it tells you and let your muscles adapt slowly to the stretch you introduced to them. Avoid overstretching, so you will not end up hurting yourself.

Required Frequency

Provided you are still in tip-top shape regardless of your age, you will have no limitations on how frequently you should perform your stretching exercises. You can do it anytime and anywhere as it is proven beneficial for anybody, regardless of age.

However, if you are a senior and are not yet used to doing stretching exercises, it would be much better to take everything slowly. Begin with basic stretches – the ones that suit beginners. Do them twice or thrice per week.

Check your comfort level as time passes. Once you begin to feel more comfortable with the stretching exercises, it may be time to increase the number of times you perform the routine every week. Do not hesitate to perform additional stretches. Perform the stretches more frequently, too. You can increase the frequency to four to five days every week.

Basically, you are allowed to stretch based on the number of times you feel inclined to do the exercise. For instance, if you sit for a prolonged period and suddenly feel some stiffness, do some basic stretches as a means of waking up your muscles. You can do the same in case you feel stressed or tense. Stretching for a few minutes can work wonders when it comes to improving your mental or emotional health.

Safety Tips for Seniors

For seniors to know that a particular stretching exercise is safe for them, they must consult their doctor first. It is also crucial for them to remember that stretching should not be a cause of pain and discomfort for them. If you are a senior, you only need to adhere to stretching instructions based on what your body can comfortably handle. The motions should never trigger any kind of pain.

Note that even if you still cannot perform full-range motion for a couple of stretches, you can still gain plenty of rewarding benefits. Eventually, you will notice your strength and flexibility improving, making it easier for you to perform the stretches. Be guided with some safety tips necessary for seniors who intend to make stretching a part of their regular routines.

- Practice deep breathing while stretching. Inhale deeply and exhale slowly, so you can maximize the effects of the stretch.

- Hold the stretch for a max of 30 seconds. This should give your muscles enough time to relax.

- Avoid bouncing when stretching as it may only result in injuries.

- Stretch only until you feel muscle tension but not extreme pain.

- Warm up before you stretch. Try to set aside around 5 to 10 minutes to move around so you can warm up your muscles. One example is taking a walk.

Safe Stretching Exercises for Seniors

The stretches covered here are safe for seniors to do. They are so safe yet effective that most seniors can do the exercises every day.

Neck Side Stretch

This is a great morning stretching routine that is ideal for seniors. The reason is that it is simple to do. It is beneficial as it loosens the tension affecting your neck and the topmost part of your shoulders. You may get this kind of tension if you sleep in an uncomfortable and incorrect position for a long time.

- Sit tall in a chair. Lean your head gently to one side.

- Raise your right arm over your head. Let your palm gently rest on the left part.

- Pull your head gently to your right. Do it as gently as possible. As a matter of fact, the simple act of putting your hand there is enough to make you feel a stretch.

- Hold this position for around 20 to 30 seconds. Repeat the steps but make sure to switch to the other side.

Upper Back and Shoulder Stretch

This stretching routine is ideal for you if your stiff back starts causing difficulties in standing up straight. The stiffness in your back may be brought on by prolonged sitting that may eventually result in your upper back and shoulders rounding forward.

Soon enough, you will find it difficult to stand straight since your muscles have become used to remaining in a hunched position. This stretching routine is a big help for seniors who experience that problem as it helps in loosening up their muscles and boosting their spinal flexibility.

- Stand tall while positioning your arms by your side.

- Swing your arms backward and behind you back.

- Pull back your shoulders while clasping your fingers behind your buttocks.

- Observe whether you already feel a stretch. If there is, hold that position. However, if you think that you can still go further, then push your clasped hands away from the lower part of your back. Arch backward gently.

- Go back to the initial standing position, then repeat the steps.

Hip Stretch

Older adults, especially women, experience some form of hip tension. If you have the same problem, you can use the hip stretch to alleviate stiffness in the area while you preserve your range of motion. Hip pain can also be prevented in older adults if they do this type of stretch regularly. Sticking into a consistent stretching routine can significantly improve your balance and mobility, thereby lowering your risk of falls and possible injuries.

- Lie on your back to stretch your hips.

- Bring one of your knees out so it can be on the side.

- Let your footrest against the opposite leg.

- Push down gently on your bent knee and continue doing so until there is a noticeable stretch.

Triceps Stretch

Building strong triceps is essential for seniors considering how these muscles are involved in every movement that your hands do. These include even precise movements like pushing and throwing heavy objects. With mobile and strong triceps, you can improve the stability of your hands.

Note that this does not necessarily mean hitting the triceps from all possible directions, volume, and intensity range, especially if you are a senior. Your goal here is to strengthen them as much as possible without putting yourself under a lot of stress or causing an injury.

The good thing about this triceps stretch is that you can choose to do it while sitting or standing and improve the mobility and flexibility in your upper back and arms as well in the process.

- Stand tall or sit in a chair.

- Raise your right arm, moving it up on top of your head. Bend at your elbow when doing so.

- Reach the left arm up so you can clasp your elbow.

- Pull it gently, moving in the opposite direction. By this time, you may start feeling light and gentle stretch in the upper arms from the back.

- Hold this pose for 20 to 30 seconds. Switch arms, then do the steps again.

Standing Quadriceps Stretch

This stretching exercise works incredibly well if you intend to lengthen your quadriceps muscles that can be found in the front of your thigh. Note that your quads tend to get tight and shortened over time because of prolonged sitting.

Hunching forward constantly may also cause tightness in your quads, further leading to poor posture and pain. You can resolve that with the help of the standing quadriceps stretch.

- Stand tall. Hold onto a countertop or back of a chair using your free hand so you can attain balance.

- Bend the right knee slowly, bring your foot toward your buttocks, then hold your foot. By this time, expect to feel a stretch at the front part of your thigh.

- Stay in this position for around 30 seconds, then do the routine again on your other leg.

If you have trouble using your hand to reach the foot, use a band or yoga strap.

Ankle Circles

The ankle circles are fantastic additions to your fitness program as a senior. Note that weak and stiff ankles can cause problems when trying to maintain your balance. You can gain greater flexibility in these areas through ankle circles.

With that, you will have a strong defense against the risk of stumbles and falls. Ankle circles also work in increasing the flow of blood through your legs. This can further prevent pooling.

- Sit up tall in a strong chair. Make sure that you are comfortable enough when you are in this starting position.

- Your right leg should then be extended in front of you. Keep the left one on the floor.

- Start rotating your right ankle. Aim to rotate it 10 to 20 times clockwise and another 10 to 20 times counterclockwise.

- Put it back down, then do the same steps with the left leg.

Forearm Stretch

Also called wrist flexion stretch, the forearm stretch is an incredible stretching routine that can greatly benefit seniors prone to injuries. This kind of stretch can help maintain your extensors and flexors' flexibility. The improved flexibility in those areas can prevent you from overusing your injuries that may cause health issues that we refer to as tendinitis and tenosynovitis.

- Sit up tall but comfortably in your chair. Bring your shoulders down and back.

- Put one of your arms directly in front of you. Your palm should face down.

- After that, allow your wrist to drop, letting it weaken.

- Bend your wrist using your other hand. Do this by applying gentle pressure to the back of your hand. Make sure that you pull your fingers and hand toward your elbow, too. Keep a straight arm during the entire stretch.

- Hold this pose for a specified period, then repeat on the other side.

The stretches here may be simple for seniors to follow, but the power you can get from them is enormous. By doing the mentioned stretches regularly, you can continue controlling your body and enjoying independence even as you age. Make them part of your daily routine, and you will surely continue to enjoy the freedom of movement. This is a good thing, as a body in motion will remain in motion.

Conclusion

Stretching is the key to improving your flexibility and restoring your mobility that may have been negatively hampered by excessive use of your muscles and body parts. It helps you let go of all the muscle tension, pain, and stress that you have been experiencing.

If you just went through an injury or suffered from a health condition that requires surgery, the best way to recover and bring back the function of the affected body part and your muscles is stretching. Fortunately, it is not that hard to make stretching a part of your life.

With the tips and tricks relevant to stretching for beginners mentioned here, you can take advantage of a wide range of stretches that will truly make your life better. Hopefully, you can use the information you have learned here to regain your confidence and the quality of your life.

Thank you for buying and reading/listening to our book. If you found this book useful/helpful please take a few minutes and leave a review on Amazon.com or Audible.com (if you bought the audio version).

References

Anusha. (2021, August 9). *Get a flexible body with ballistic stretching and improve your fitness*. Activeman.Com. https://activeman.com/ballistic-stretching/

ASFA. (n.d.). *Active vs. Passive stretching – know the difference!* Americansportandfitness.Com. Retrieved from https://www.americansportandfitness.com/blogs/fitness-blog/active-vs-passive-stretching-know-the-difference

Ava English, J. T. (2021, April 21). *9 of the best static stretches to improve flexibility, posture, and mobility*. Insider.Com; Insider. https://www.insider.com/static-stretching

Ballistic stretching types, disadvantages & how ballistic stretching is done. (2019, February 11). Healthjade.Net. https://healthjade.net/ballistic-stretching/

Bass, L. (2021, July 15). *Active stretching: Definition, benefits, exercises to try*. Greatist.Com; Greatist. https://greatist.com/fitness/active-stretching

Blackwell, R. (n.d.). *Why stretching is important in active aging and functional training*. Hurusa.Com. Retrieved from https://blog.hurusa.com/why-stretching-is-important-in-active-aging-and-functional-training

Boland, W. M. (2016, October 24). *Flexibility vs. Mobility: The Differences Between Them & How To Make Them Work Together*. Bodyfixmethod.Com. https://www.bodyfixmethod.com/flexibility-vs-mobility-differences-make-work-together/

Cronkleton, E. (2019, October 17). *How long to hold a stretch, how often and best time to stretch*. Healthline.Com. https://www.healthline.com/health/how-long-to-hold-a-stretch

Crowley, K. (2020, September 7). *Is flexibility important? 5 reasons why stretching is good for you*. Gymondo.Com. https://www.gymondo.com/magazin/en/workout/is-flexibility-important-5-reasons-why-stretching-is-good-for-you

de Grasse, M. (2021, September 14). *Static Stretching: What is it and when should you do it?* Energy.Fit; www.energy.fit. https://www.energy.fit/blogs/news/static-stretching

Elkaim, Y. (2017, February 14). *9 important stretching exercises for seniors to do every day*. Yurielkaim.Com. https://yurielkaim.com/stretching-exercises-seniors

Ferraro, K. (2021, March 24). *How to start A stretching routine, according to fitness pros*. Bustle.Com; Bustle. https://www.bustle.com/wellness/how-to-start-a-stretching-routine-fitness-experts/amp

Fitness, C. (2018, April 9). *Dynamic stretching: What is it and when should I do it?* Chuzefitness.Com. https://chuzefitness.com/blog/dynamic-stretching-what-is-it-and-how-do-you-do-it/

Flexibility vs. Mobility: What's the difference? (2017, August 7). Precisionmovement.Coach. https://www.precisionmovement.coach/flexibility-vs-mobility/

healtheloo. (2020, January 3). *Ballistic Stretching Benefits And Exercises*. Healtheloo.Com. https://healtheloo.com/ballistic-stretching-benefits/

How often and how long to stretch. (n.d.). Easyflexibility.Com. Retrieved from https://www.easyflexibility.com/blogs/flexibility-pearls/how-often-and-how-long-to-stretch

Kelly, D. R. (2020, May 5). *The importance of stretching and flexibility*. Studymartialarts.Org. https://www.studymartialarts.org/blog/the-importance-of-stretching-and-flexibility

Kutcher, M. (2019, July 1). *Regaining Flexibility After 60.*
Morelifehealth.Com; More Life Health - Seniors Health &
Fitness. https://morelifehealth.com/articles/regaining-
flexibility-guide

News. (2020, July 15). *5 passive stretching exercises that can
reduce muscle stiffness and heart disease risk.* News18.
https://www.news18.com/news/lifestyle/passive-stretching-
exercises-myupchar-2717679.html

Panchal, B. (n.d.). *The benefits of dynamic stretching.*
Hollandandbarrett.Com. Retrieved from
https://www.hollandandbarrett.com/the-health-
hub/conditions/bone-joint-muscle-health/the-benefits-of-
dynamic-stretching/

podium. (2017, September 1). *Ten static stretching exercises.*
Newcastlesportsinjury.Co.Uk.
https://www.newcastlesportsinjury.co.uk/ten-static-
stretching-exercises/

Pt, L.-A. B., DPT, EdD, & COMT. (n.d.). *Static vs. Dynamic
stretching: What are they and which should you
do?* Hss.Edu. Retrieved from
https://www.hss.edu/article_static_dynamic_stretching.asp

Sita. (2020, July 24). *What is Flexibility vs Range of Motion.*
Bendablebody.Com. https://bendablebody.com/what-is-
flexibility-vs-range-of-motion/

Stretching and flexibility: 7 tips. (n.d.-a). Webmd.Com. Retrieved from https://www.webmd.com/fitness-exercise/features/stretching-and-flexibility-tips

Stretching and flexibility: 7 tips. (n.d.-b). Webmd.Com. Retrieved from https://www.webmd.com/fitness-exercise/features/stretching-and-flexibility-tips

The benefits of dynamic stretching and how to get started. (2021, September 7). Bigandripped.Com. https://bigandripped.com/benefits-of-dynamic-stretching/

The dos and don'ts of stretching. (n.d.). Healthyfamiliesbc.Ca. Retrieved from https://www.healthyfamiliesbc.ca/home/blog/dos-and-donts-stretching

Todd Kuslikis, H. I. L. (2015, August 3). *Isometric exercises: 7 moves for your shoulders, abs, legs, and more*. Greatist.Com; Greatist. https://greatist.com/move/isometric-exercises

Types of stretches. (2016, January 4). Thepeakperformancecenter.Com. https://thepeakperformancecenter.com/athletics/physical-development/flexibility/types-of-stretches/

Types of Stretching. (n.d.-a). Acefitness.Org. Retrieved from https://www.acefitness.org/fitness-certifications/ace-answers/exam-preparation-blog/2966/types-of-stretching/

Types of Stretching. (n.d.-b). Mit.Edu. Retrieved from
https://web.mit.edu/tkd/stretch/stretching_4.html

UAB Medicine News. (n.d.). Uabmedicine.Org. Retrieved from
https://www.uabmedicine.org/-/starting-a-stretching-
routine-do-s-and-don-ts

What is static stretching? (2009, September 29). Projectswole.Com.
https://www.projectswole.com/flexibility/what-is-static-
stretching/

Wilke, K. (2015, October 3). *The horrifying consequences of not
stretching.* Outwardon.Com.
https://outwardon.com/article/the-horrifying-consequences-
of-not-stretching/

(N.d.-a). Bereact.Com. Retrieved from
https://www.bereact.com/the-benefits-of-ballistic-stretching/

(N.d.-b). Healthgrades.Com. Retrieved from
https://www.healthgrades.com/right-care/bones-joints-and-
muscles/10-stretching-dos-and-donts

(N.d.-c). Fitnessvigil.Com. Retrieved from
https://fitnessvigil.com/passive-vs-active-stretching

Table of Contents

WAX OIL WOMEN

EROTICA ROMANCE

J KINFOLK

This book is a work of fiction. The author uses their imagination to depict all the characters, organizations, and events in this novel.

The publisher requires prior written permission for reproducing, storing, or transmitting any part of this publication in any form or by any means, electronic, mechanical, photocopying, recording, or otherwise.

Synopsis

Thaddeus Kofi was all for providing a healing effect for those who had been wounded. He was not one for turning anyone away however he did have some boundaries. Opening a new establishment he was also wanting to fill the empty void in his life. With the use of oils, candles, music he would become what all women craved. Thaddeus "Magic " Kofi of Majestic Massage Spa is your sensual massage masseuse.

When heartache finds you, it's either you sit back and take it or you give it some push back. The second option is what Sunny Dalton did, pushing back was not in her vocabulary. A go with the flow person is what got her almost on the wrong side of love. To recover was her goal, by any means necessary.

Sunny made herself a checklist of Moving out of Stuck with a Hot Girl, Act Bad, Bald-Headed Hoe, FNF amongst other songs to get her way back to herself. To add fuel to the fire it took no prisoners for her.

Come inside while these pages unfold how both Sunny and Thaddeus worlds collide in a special way. They will not disappoint

Chapter 1

The sun was working its way high into the sky illuminating another beautiful summer morning in the city. It was the final day for the AMT (American Massage Therapy) convention, the view we had from the hotel overlooked the skyline on one side and the beautiful lake on the other. This trip was what Thaddeus needed to push my business to the next level. Opening up my own spa had been a dream; however life had dealt me the perfect opportunity after a ten-year breakup. The hurt, and betrayal with the push from my cousin Nathan and best friend Rodney.

"Thaddeus !!!! Thaddeus !!!! Come on, we need to leave, so we can finish this final seminar." Rodney, his business partner, and friend was telling him.

"Alright!! I'm coming, just getting my mind right." Thaddeus responded.

Thaddeus and Rodney began to head out towards the lobby to get the day started.

Thaddeus is what you would call a good catch, one of a few men that is left of his caliber. At thirty years old, about 6'3" tall, he is very muscular with an athletic build with black well styled dreads. Thaddeus now is single, no kids, his own home, and a new business owner. One day he wanted to have a family, however that went up in flames after the betrayal of his ex-girlfriend Gina. The way Thaddeus had thrown himself into his work and potential family was priceless. It's now all about making himself happy at any cost. The time he spent in college learning his trade was about to pay off. The business classes he took on the side as well as the hands-on experience from his cousin Nathan, a business owner himself. Thaddeus remembered back when he was getting into the massage business he was teased that his hands would one day be lethal.

After the guys finished the final class it was time to see what the town had in store for them on their last night in town. Thaddeus headed to his room to shower and prepare for the night, but not until he began to check his calendar for this shop. Just before he left he had opened a slot for sensual intimate massages, as a request he had from one of his clients. The professional way managed his business was highly spoken of; he serviced those who needed a simple massage to be more detailed, in a private space. Thaddeus' eyes widened to see how many sensual massages he had on his calendar for the upcoming weeks. The trying information he obtained from this convention will definitely come in handy as he was flipping through his calendar.

"D'uesse with a side of coke," Thaddeus called out to the bartender, while he and Rodney decided to hang out on their last night at the convention. The music was popping as they glanced at the crowd in the far corner of the club. There was a beautiful woman that seemed to be enjoying herself. Thaddeus was mesmerized by her beauty.

"Oh I see you, go ahead and say something, we are going to be here for another twenty-four hours. Make it a memorable one." Rodney was stating while he also noticed how his friend had drifted off staring at the woman.

Finally Thaddeus made his way over to the young lady after our eyes had met. The attraction was instant as we began to stare each other down. Thaddeus walked over to her introducing himself.

"Hello, how are you? Would you like another drink or some water?" he asked while standing over top of this young woman. She responded with a yes as he motioned the bartender to bring over the both of them another drink.

"He wasn't going to ask why such a beautiful woman is sitting alone in a bar. He thought he could figure it out but why assume when you can just tell me." Thaddeus asked the beautiful woman.

She opened her mouth speaking to me stating that she was in town for a seminar on business. The two of them talked for another thirty minutes until they ended up going to ten more flirty conversations. Thaddeus was at his wits of how much he wanted to have this woman for himself. In the back of his mind he thought of some of those moves he learned in the convention. With that last bold statement Thaddeus stated, "Well I'm only in town for tonight..."

"Well that works for me, your room or mine." The beautiful woman stated. It was a surreal moment the two who were strangers will no longer be once they got behind closed doors. Smiles on both of their faces not knowing what to expect from each other.

Thaddeus stood up from the table leaving a few bills on it, He reached out for her hand and then led her outside where they shared an Uber to his hotel. Thaddeus was staying at the convention hotel so it was closer to the club. The drive was silent until the driver pulled up and they exited. Taddeus led her to his room, opening the door, only to have her attack his mouth with hers. She was aggressive unlike what he was accounted for, in a sexy way. Each moment was intense as their lips locked; she had wrapped her arms around his neck. Thaddeus welcomed each moment with a breeze, he led her to the bed. Without warning the two had torn each other's clothes off, Thaddeus dripped down low to taste her, thinking if she tasted as good as she looked. He began to flick his tongue as he assaulted her center to her clit. It was more than what he imagined. The shaking that he felt from her legs almost wrapping around his neck had him smiling. Thaddeus was experienced but this was different for him.

Thaddeus wasn't much of a kisser but with her he kissed her passionately after experiencing how delicious she tasted. The way she moaned in his mouth sent him over the top, he was ready to put in some work on her. The way he mounted her and began to fill her up with his enormous length. Thaddeus was blown away as he began to stroke her with first short pounds to only begin to do long deep strokes. The warmth he felt from her insides was priceless. Thaddeus thought to himself, he knew he wasn't a minute man but this felt sooooo good.

"oohhh you're so tight and warm," he moaned in her ear while on top of her. When he couldn't take anymore he exploded deep inside of her walls. Unable to contain his emotions Thaddeus rolled off of her, only to be surprised by her taking his dick in her hands to massage it back to a perfect erection. This young woman had him feeling like he was in his early twenties. The way she massaged his penis, then taking him in her mouth had his eyes rolling in the back of his head. The night had been long but turned short as he rolled his eyes in the back of his head. The pleasure he experienced was priceless. It was the final round that both Thaddeus and the young lady spent. He didn't realize that he was not the lead in tonight's intense love making. It was great for someone to meet him intimately and to actually keep up. To his reality the night was perfect he thought, the time he spent at the convention and with this young lady didn't owe him anything.

It was early morning when Thaddeus heard his alarm going off letting him know it was time to get up. The wake time he requested was for another two hours but Thaddeus noticed Rodney had texted him stating the request for an early flight was approved. It. At that moment he regretted wanting to leave earlier, he hadn't anticipated that he would meet someone. Taking the short strides towards the bathroom, Thaddeus was moving like a turtle, he got his hygiene together, packed all his bags to leave. Thaddeus looked over in the bed to see the sleeping beauty still resting.

There were no names they had shared; he took upon himself to write her a note saying what a great time he had. Thaddeus took that moment to leave her with his business card as well. This would be a memory that he didn't want to forget. Shaking his head assuring the room was intact he left out heading to the airport.

"Hey man, we got lucky to get on this early flight together," Rodney had stated, looking at his best friend. "Oh no what is it, you got that look."

"You are right my brother I didn't want to leave just yet. Last night wasn't long enough, it was a new beginning for me. Something I didn't expect." Thaddeus was telling his best friend. "I'm so glad that we came to this convention."

"Well we can get back and hopefully what happened last night can continue on into the future." Rodney was trying to give him some hope. Thaddeus was sure it should when he left his card with the beauty that was laying in his hotel bed. The smile that landed on his face was priceless as him and Rodney boarded the plane. Both the men got to their seats and enjoyed their flight back home.

Chapter 2

Sunny sat up in the bed looking around in a daze, her head throbbing from the multiple Sangria's she drank last night. Her body ached, in a not too pleasant way, from the intense activity from last night in a good way. Taking in her surroundings Sunny knew she wasn't in her room, but the handsome stranger who was gone. Holy Shit she shouted she immediately went into a panic, which soon faded with memories of last night.

Here I am sitting on the side of the bed, which is huge, a perfect fit for the handsome guy I was with last night. I gathered up my clothes and headed to the bathroom to freshen up. There was a note on the mirror.

Had a great time last night, you are amazing. Red eye flight, stay as long as you want the check-out is noon.

The note was attached to a business card, with all his information on it. Thaddeus Kofi, she said his name like a hundred times in my mind. Snapping back to the current, my hair was all over the place. My body ached in some places that I thought didn't exist. Sunny get it together girl, you should be ashamed of yourself. She was giving herself a pep talk.

"Hello?" she answered.

"Sunny, are you alright? What the hell, I called you last night like five times and texted you three." Lynn was talking a mile a minute to her cousin.

"Calm down girl, you are worse than my momma. I'm alive but girl I have some tea for you." Sunny stated. "Give me another thirty minutes to call you so I can spill it girl."

Sunny had arrived at her hotel to get prepared for her departure herself. Slipping on her fatigue tights, with her signature banded t-shirt, the best relief was the camo Nike that she loved topped with a baseball cap.

The check out process was easy, as Sunny made her way to the hotel shuttle heading to the airport. With her bags now checked in the monitors showed her flight had been delayed for another hour. What better time to call her cousin she thought remembering that she wanted to vent to someone. Sunny dialed the number, within the first two rings Lynn answers.

"Dang girl what took you so long, I thought I was going to have to come get you." Lynn teased.

"Cousin," Sunny whined, " Where did she begin, it's so much this weekend was everything. From the time she arrived at the resort, the staff for the seminar was so nice. It was five-star treatment from the time she had accepted the invitation as speaker." Sunny began going on and on about the seminar until Lynn cut her off.

"Nawl heifer get to the meat, cause if you keep going about that get your mind right seminar I'm hanging up. What happened to that loser, Myron, showed up on you. Did you get your back blown out by some headliner?" Lynn was hounding for information that she knew was unlike another.

"Girl shut up, really a Headliner, just be my luck she was being catfished. That abusive loser Myron knows not to show up on me. I'll exercise my restraining order of two thousand square feet on him. I may even use my taser to show him I mean business." They both laughed.

Sunny had been in a controlling, abusive relationship with her ex-Myron for almost five years. It was hard for her to imagine that they would ever break up. He was with her during some rough patches in life only to try and control her every move. When Sunny was accepted as a panelist for a prestige podcast, he was jealous. Her love of fashion was perfect for her personality. Immediately after her four shows, the request for her to travel for speaking engagements was too much for Myron he felt left out. The mental, emotional, and eventually physical abuse started. Sunny was glad to get out when she did. Now free of that life she had taken Lynn up on her constant nagging to live your life to the fullest. Little did Lynn now this past weekend Sunny did just that as she began to spill the tea.

"What! You didn't, girl." Lynn was listening to the details as if Sunny were sitting in front of her.

"Yes, cousin. I was the original Sunny Sunshine, pulled out all tricks and then some. Lynn was amazing, the conversations were limited to almost none. Our chemistry was like we had been together for years. He allowed me to be free, take charge and he loved it." Sunny gave her some graphic explanations. "Lynn, the man almost blacked out from these Gawk 3000 skills I put on him. If bald headed hoe shit was a person it was me." Sunny started cracking up at her own jokes. "Yes I actually enjoyed the one night, with Mr. Handsome girl, truly enjoyed it."

"So when are you going to see him again? she asked if she had made plans yet to see him." Lynn asked. The silence lasted too long for her likings. "Sunny, Sunny are you there?"

"Yes, I'm here girl. The thought of my hoe status just registered; I had my first one-night stand." Sunny confessed. "Bitch I loved it! There is just one thing, he doesn't know my name, he left his business card."

While the trip was business, it was good that Sunny had time to unwind and enjoy herself. It was what Lynn had told her she needed, but never that she would be a one-night stand kind of girl. They both address the issue of Sunny relocating in another few weeks to be closer to her family. While at least to be closer to Lynn and her daughter since they had been so close. Sunny would also be able to see her parents more being on the west coast had been too much. So moving back to the east coast was what she needed.

"Well she also called to let you know your condo is ready, it is beautiful. It overlooks the city and the stadium. This was prize real estate; you got a deal, girl." Lynn explained she had done all the necessary tasks to make sure her cousin moved in smoothly.

"Thank you so much, for being my favorite cousin." Sunny was grateful for Lynn; she helped her so much, the same as when Lynn was in need at one time. "Did you let Natalie decorate her room?" Sunny waited until she finished to brag on how she couldn't wait to move so she could spoil Lynn's daughter.

"Yes, she used all the swatches and pictures you and she discussed too. You will be pleased at how her little four-year-old mind put it all together." Lynn explained then got back to the one question she wanted to ask Sunny. "So when are you going to call this guy? He seems to be a nice gentleman,

"They are calling me to board the plane now, I'll be in touch when I get ready to come into town for good. I love you cousin." Sunny stated as she hung up the phone heading to the gate to board her plane.

Once Sunny returned home she had so much she had to consider making decisions to change her life. The first one was when she stepped out to start her own business, the breakup with her ex. Then to challenge herself with the speaking engagement that she did in Vegas. Most people wouldn't have done that, instead would have just had a pity party. Sunny took the world by the horns, did what she wanted to do without any regrets.

After talking to her cousin, she didn't feel guilty about doing a one-night stand, it was her life and she was in charge of it. No longer a victim to anyone else. Sunny knew her mother would be proud of her for doing what she wanted to do, not what everyone else thought she should be doing. Thinking to herself she laughed, "momma would you sleep with a guy on the first night?" she could hear her mother say, "Girl, she would get back shots, throw it around in a circle. ride him like a cowgirl from the back" those conversations she missed having with her mother. They had a strained relationship once Sunny had moved away and cut off most of her family. What she would give to have one of those feisty conversations with her mom. Sunny had to place on her agenda to send her mother an email in the near future, until then it's her and her cousin Lynn for now.

Now that Sunny made the choice to relocate closer to family, she had a few loose ends to tie up. Sitting at her old office for the last time, Sunny took out the business card that Thaddeus Kofi, the Magic Masseuse had given her. She wanted to call him, knowing that they shared more than just a few drinks. Sunny could still feel that ultimate pleasure that he gave to her in Vegas. The things she did were not from a textbook, Sunny wanted to try plenty of those porn hubs and XXX video moves she saw without judgment. That night she was able to deliver just that, Thaddeus didn't know who she was and wouldn't be able to look at her any differently the next day or week. That was one of the pluses for going to Vegas, as they would say what goes on in Vegas stays in Vegas.

Sunny dialed the number on the card, before she could follow through she hung up placing the card back into her bag. The way her nerves just triggered had her ready to pass out. It was the effect that he had on her just in the one encounter. When there was almost a full ring she got nervous having heart palpitations, palms sweating, and her throat felt like it was about to close. For the first time in a while this feeling hadn't happened to Sunny, she thought she was a kid in school, calling a new boy. What kind of foolishness she thought was happening to her. Sunny's inner thoughts got the best of her, so Sunny made a mental note to herself to call her cousin to talk about it again. Now she was going to pack her things to prepare for her big move.

Chapter 3

"Welcome to Majestic Massage and Spa, please follow me this way." Samantha the receptionist led one of the clients towards the lobby. It was the grand opening of the hottest spa in the art district. Once the woman was seated Samantha paged her boss to inform him that his next appointment was here. The lobby was crowned as the clients waited for their turn to experience the well-known hands of the staff at Majestic. The buzz around town was that you can stop in to get a wonderful massage from the best-looking masseuse in the area. It was an upscale atmosphere that delivered the best quality service.

"Thank you Karen, you can see Samantha for your next appointment." Thaddeus was walking towards the receptionist area when he noticed the waiting area was full. It was just as he had anticipated after announcing the additional services for the sensual massages. He had made his business the main priority for him. Looking over the books he noticed he had three more appointments for the day one being a full-service sensual massage. The way he felt about being a man of pleasure made him smile. Although there were no strings attached he felt a sense of peace. It was like a healing from the pain he had experienced in the past. Hearing his name being called Thaddeus snapped back, to reply to Samantha. "Yes Sam, send in my next client."

For the next forty minutes Thaddeus had his client on his table as he played some music and lit up the candles that were in the room that was used for this type of massage. Greeting his client he began to explain what he would be doing in accordance to her request from the form she completed.

"So are you ready? It shows you have had this kind of massage in the past, is that correct?" Thaddeus had to make sure no gaps were left in the paperwork, he assured that he would say she signed the NDA. That was something that he learned at the convention a few months ago. This business could lead to some legal issues if he wasn't careful. With a final glance over the paperwork Thaddeus began his work.

"Yesss, that's it," was the one sign from the young lady that he was doing what he had been trained to do. She was not new to the massaging techniques that were being used, he could tell. The more he began to work his hands into her soft skin made the task easy. Thaddeus took his thumb and began to rub it across her nipples; she began to tremble from his touch. The music was soothing for him as he continued to work his way down to her belly button, to her shaved mound. The sexual essence filled the air; almost to an extent of overpowering the candles he had lit in the room. This was another tell sign that he was bringing more than relaxation but of pleasure to his client. "I'm about to touch your thighs," Thaddeus explained his next moves would be intense for her to let him know If she felt uncomfortable.

"I'm perfectly fine," she stated as she let out a quiet moan." That was more than enough for Thaddeus to go ahead and deliver that for which she paid. He slid the condom down on his ten inches, it was just another day at the office for him, the self-control he had come natural from the meditation and yoga he practiced daily. Thaddeus was thankful for his strength in this area, most women loved a man with stamina. He was glad to be able to use it to his advantage.

"Oohhh shit," escaped from the woman's mouth, the strokes that he delivered would bring any woman to a climax. Thaddeus used all his strength to do just what he was paid to do. To work out areas that she hadn't used in a while, bringing a release that would be more relaxing than imagined. Within the next five minutes he did that with his fingers and his dick. Giving her slow to fast strokes pounding deep inside of her walls.

"Hello, you are done." He had to wake her up, she had fallen into a deep sleep after her fifth orgasm. Once he finished the sensual massage she was more than relaxed, which she expressed to him as she prepared to leave.

"Mr. Magic, thank you I will be sure to schedule a follow up in the next thirty days." The woman was completely satisfied with the services that were delivered.

Hi Melissa, Thaddeus greeted his final customer for the day. There was no routine for them, Mellissa was his regular girl currently. The two of them had an understanding that it's just sex, he was clear that nothing would ever come of what they had going on.

Once back in his room that he used for the tantra massages, Melissa immediately went down on her knees to take Thaddeus in her mouth. He just watched as she tried to obtain a reaction from him. It was not that she wasn't doing a good job, he was just not into her that way. Thaddeus was okay with her getting him prepared to take her loose vagina. He went ahead and pretended that she was doing a great job, with the simply dry moan he threw at her. "Mmmm do that shit," he said. "You ready for me to pound that ass."

Melissa was always ready; she had a wet pussy but it was not what he would call wife material. Thaddeus placed a condom on his erect penis then slid up into Melissa. The thoughts of the mystery woman came into his mind, it had him going in hard and rough. It was when Melissa screamed out his name that brought him back to see her face with tears running down her cheek. "Damn, Thaddeus what was that about? You have never been like that with me." Melissa was stating, as she began to put her clothes back on after wiping herself down. "Is it something you need to tell me, Thaddeus?"

He was looking at her like she had two heads as he stated, "You know what time it is with us, Melissa, we aren't in a relationship this is just sex nothing more. If I was too rough then we can chill on anything else moving forward." Melissa was hurt and she showed that she had begun to care more than just sex with Thaddeus.

"Hey, I'm packing up for the night when my day is done. You were my last client." Rolling her eyes she left out without saying goodbye.

Thaddeus was happy that he was doing well, when he turned to go into his office he had no other appointments left for the day. Sitting at his desk he was trying to decide if he was going to go over to his cousins club when a page came to his phone. It was from Samantha asking him to squeeze in a walk in that Rodney had forgotten about. It appeared he overbooked once again. That was the only thing about being a business owner that he had to remember he is the brand to his company so it would take him to cover when things may happen if he could. Without hesitation or just a small moment he thought of Melissa prior to taking this next client.

The young woman was happy to see that she was going to be able to get her in. Samantha sent Thaddeus a thank you and to inform him that she was leaving for the day.

"Come this way, I'm Magic and I'll be helping you today with your massage." Thaddeus wasn't sure what was requested just yet but he made sure to give her his best.

"Thank you, I'm Nicole, your company was referred to me by a coworker that comes here often. I had an accident a few months ago that my insurance stopped paying so a readjustment is exactly what I need to my shoulder." She was rambling on about his needs while Thaddeus was reading over her card, when he got to the services he noticed she checked the vaginal tantra massage as well as the deep tissue shoulder massage.

"Nicole, you check multiple boxes. Are you sure this is what you want? I want to assure you that you are clear, since the NDA wasn't signed." He went over the services along with the required documents that hadn't yet to be signed.

"Yes, I'm sure you came to get me before I was able to complete the final pages." Reaching for the documents she signed them and handed them back to Thaddeus with a smile. He looked her in her eyes, while she looked familiar he didn't say much more but kept it professional.

With the music playing from his exotic playlist Thaddeus proceeded to begin his massage. Nicolee was a talker; she began talking then signing to the music then she continued to talk to Thaddeus as he was doing just as she requested. The oils he used on her shoulder he could tell that she eventually relaxed to allow him to work in the areas she was tensed the most. He began to explain to her the touching and places he would be going for her vaginal massage.

Thaddus used his hands to begin on her inner thighs working his way up to the opening of her vagina entrance. Using his thumb he circled around her clit then he used a few fingers to open her up to continue working his way inside her walls. Thaddeus wasn't surprised when he felt her releasing all over his fingers. It was only two that he had slowly glided into her, the entrance was wide enough that he used four fingers. Gently working her muscles he was about to come to the end of the massage when she asked, "Can I get the full treatment please, it's been almost six months since I've had the real thing."

Clearing his throat, Thaddeus' eyes got wide as he wasn't prepared for that statement. She had already signed the NDA and he wouldn't want to disappoint the client so he motioned for her to sit up and come to the edge of the table. Pulling her into his body as he positioned her lower body then leaned her into him. Thaddeus placed a condom over himself to assure nothing would be missed. He gently slid himself into her, causing her to release a slow moan into his neck. Each stroke he gave she received with no problem. Thaddeus took his large hands and guided her hips while massaging into her inner thighs. He knew she was about to explode on his dick when he felt her breathing pick up and she thrust into him forcefully. He had to tell her to relax, or she wouldn't get the complete relief she was looking for.

"Right there doesn't stop, it feels so good. I'm about to cum," is the last words he heard from her as she moaned in his ear. That was it for him, again not one time did Thaddeus relieve himself but assured his clients were satisfied.

Once Nicole was dressed, he escorted her to the front to settle her tab. He thanked her as he noticed she had already scheduled another appointment with Rodney for next month, but not before giving Thaddeus a generous tip.

Chapter 4

The music was blasting loud as Thaddeus, Rodney and their coworker Charlie walked into the Temptation's Den club. It had been over two months since the three had come back from the convention getting back to the swing of things. Rodney was still asking Thaddeus about his hook up prior to leaving Las Vegas, knowing the code of what goes on in Vegas stays in Vegas. It was just the vibes that Thaddeus had given was saying he wanted to talk about the beauty that he encountered.

"So spill it Thaddeus you've been acting real weird since we got back from the convention please tell me what happened," Rodney was grilling his best friend since he knew the downward hole he had once seen him in. The way he was acting lately had him concerned. Rodney told Thaddeus, "I let you slide long enough, so you got to give me all the tea." Rondey was leaning in towards his friend.

"No, I'm cool just trying to keep my focus on getting this money." Thaddeus replied with a smirk on his face. He had been scanning the crowd looking for his victim to put on his list of victims in his hit and quit it. Outside of his job getting his dick wet was his motto, not to have any feeling for these women in the streets. Rodney did hit a nerve asking about the mystery woman whom he didn't get her name from. What Thaddeus did remember was her beautiful smile along with her scent of essence that she had. It wasn't of any fragrance; it was a natural scent of pineapple, and sage; when he knew that everyone had a scent to make them unique. Making his way over to the bar again he got himself and Rodney another drink. Thaddeus had the eerie feeling that someone was staring at him, so he turned around scanning the crowd again.

When Thaddeus got back over to the table he thought someone was watching him. When Rodney asked him again about his wild night in Vegas Thaddeus said, "It was the most exciting night of my life, it was heaven. The way we express ourselves intimately was like we belonged together. I felt like she could be the one. I never got her name either, she has my card." The burn in his gut was felt when he even tried to say what he felt or wanted to try to put a name to her face. The way she rode his face, the way she rode his dick made him wear a smile that couldn't be erased.

Both Rodney and Nate looked at Thaddeus like he had two heads. While they both knew the pain that Thaddeus had suffered behind his last break up so happiness was something they wanted for him.

"So she hadn't called you yet?" Rodney asked, without thinking. Nate noticed his girl walking in when he told them he would catch them later. Just before he walked off he told Thaddeus to keep his head up as the old saying what is meant to be will be.

The music was playing as a few of the latest summer hits blurred through the speakers, the thoughts of the night spent in Vegas as on the forefront of Thaddues mind. He noticed a familiar face walking over towards him when he started to smile until it was Melissa who he wasn't expecting to see tonight. In the side view he saw Rodney laughing knowing that Thaddeus had told her to back off, it's just sex only.

"Hey guys, I'm going to run to the restroom, I'll be back," Thaddeus stated.

"Sure man, I see my girl over there, see you both in a few." Nate told Thaddeus and Rodney.

Inside the restroom after handling his business, Thaddeus thought he saw Melissa in the crowd so he was going back out to try and dodge her to get home after he came in to just clear his mind, which was crowded with thoughts from his trip to Vegas. The convention was helpful but his last night of pleasure was unforgettable. Leaving out of the restroom Thaddeus managed to bump into another one of his clients that he had enjoyed a full night of pleasure with once. He knew that being at the Temptation Den it wouldn't be easy to not see someone he had on his rooster of women. They all knew that he was a dangerous man, not to be taken seriously. Thaddeus always made that clear that he wasn't looking for any kind of relationship to commit to only a good sexual time. That was the rules only business never pleasure when it came to him serving up some good D. Now ever since he returned from the convention, with the encounter of the beautiful woman who owns his heart he was getting his life on track. Thaddeus had caught himself thinking of a future with a family again.

"Hey, guys I'm going to run now," Thaddeus said to his friend. "I had my fix, now let me get out of here before I take some extra baggage home." The guys laughed knowing what he meant when he said that . He didn't want to know how but he was coming up with a plan to sneak out of the building not to run into Melissa nor did he want to get noticed by Gwen.

"Alright, my man," Rodney said as he two got up to leave. "I'm walking out with you too, it's my signal to leave."

The men made it out clear, getting into their separate vehicles to leave for their homes. Thaddeus was bumping his new summer playlist of songs that got into a relaxed mood, only to be sidetracked with happy thoughts of life. He got into his home, handled his hygiene, and began to do some thinking of new options that would be ahead. Pouring himself another night cap he then began to drift off to sleep to face the next day.

Chapter 5

Sunny was settled in her condo for a few weeks, she was feeling happier than ever. This move was what needed a change in the demographics. The music was blasting thru her speakers while she made some final decorating to her place. Today she was meeting with a new client for a gig. Sunny did interior design on the side along with her public speaking gigs for empowering girls and women.

"Hello, Lynn, call me when you get this message." Sunny had called her cousin to let her know she would be ready around eight so that they could go together to the club.

With Sunny being an interior designer her job could be worked remote, she loved it. Since coming into town she had a gig already to decorate an upscale hair salon. The client was extremely picky, with a beer budget with champagne taste. The video call that was about to start in less than twenty minutes had Sunny second thinking about this gig.

"Hi, I'm Sunny with Sensational Design, I have the samples ready for you to view also I've emailed them to you." The woman on the other end of the phone was just staring at Sunny for about ten seconds when she finally responded.

"Hello, Sunny it's great to get a face behind the brand, the photo on your page doesn't do you any justice girl. You are beautiful. I'm the owner of Missy's Hair Extravaganza." The two just chatted while making some final decisions on the gig.

Sunny was pleased that Missy accepted the ideas since it fit into the budget that she was given. The call ended on a good note as Sunny then prepared for her evening with her cousin.

It's about time you got here girl, we are going to have a wonderful time. Lynn was telling Sunny that her baby daddy owned the spot they were heading to so I would be all expenses on him.

"Lynn, you are too many girls, so why do you do that man this way?" Sunny was grilling Lynn because she knew that Lynn wasn't into him as she should have been. Who has a baby by their best friend and ignores him. That is an entire storyline in itself.

"Hush girl," Lynn stated, "Nathan and I have been best friends since middle school. It was a mutual understanding that she gave him my virginity before going off to London." Lynn was sure that she didn't love Nathan, but it was written all in her face.

"Why are you trying to change the subject, you still haven't called the guy from Vegas yet huh?" Sunny tried to change the subject again but Lynn wasn't having it.

"Let's make a small wager on this situation." Lynn asked. "I'll give Nathan a full chance if you call him within the next twenty-four hours."

Sunny rolled her eyes, as they were pulling up to the club. "Nice name for this spot." Lynn laughed as her wager was ignored.

"Alright it's on." Sunny smiled; she had a comeback. "When I call you will not only give him a chance but you will give him some of that desert coochie."

"Girl bye," Lynn laughed

When Lynn pulled up to the club she used the valet parking, it was their night to unwind and enjoy good music, some dancing, the food, and drinks.

"Girl, that song has got to be played on every hip hop station in the country." Lynn said as the Sexy Redd song Pound Town sounded off in the speakers. The ladies went over to the bar where the bartender recognized Lynn and got their order quickly.

"Here you go, your tab is already established," he stated. "Oh boss man said you have VIP section 8." With a wink and smile Lynn led Sunny towards the designated section. That was her favorite area of the club. It gave access to all angles, from the entrance, the bar, the dance floor, the entryway to the bathroom etc.

The night was going great when Lynn and Sunny finished dancing to their favorite songs. They stood looking over the railing to see who was in the crowd. Sunny thought she saw Mr. Thaddeus in the flow of the crowd. She was half a bottle in the Cosmigos tequila, when she whispered to Lynn, "I'm going down to the bathroom."

What Lynn didn't know is that she had indeed spotted her hot one-night stand.

Sunny had finished up in the restroom walking out and she was heading over toward the area where she saw Thaddeus standing. "Bingo" she said as she strolled over towards him.

The knowing fragrance hit her nose, it was one that she would not forget, the scent of Gucci Envy. If she was honest, the dress she had on that night still hadn't washed it yet. The scent of Thaddeus was how she would get to sleep when she had a rough day. Smelling his cologne off of the dress made her relax and most of all kept her juices flowing in her center, although it was the real thing it helped her release some stress. Sunny eased up on him to tap his shoulder when she almost fell into him. "Hi" she said while leaning inward to him.

Thaddeus turned around to catch the falling Sunny into his arms.

"Well, hello beautiful," Thaddeus said. "I'd take an in person contact over a phone call any day." Sunny was just staring into his eyes the tone of his voice with his intoxicating smell. Her panties were wet immediately, bringing back a tone of memories.

"Beautiful, what is your name? You won't get away from me this time without me getting that from you." Thaddeus smiled.

"My name is Sunny, it's nice to officially meet you Thaddeus." She smiled at him as he wrapped his arm around her waist. Sunny asked for him to follow her to let her tell her cousin that she was leaving. He followed her to the VIP, while staring at her the entire time. It was like Thaddeus was in a dream. His mystery woman, and her mystery man. The two were both gliding towards the VIP room.

In the VIP was Sunny's cousin, who was eyeing the handsome guy that followed her cousin into the section. Lynn was giving Sunny a raised eyebrow, like who is this fine man. Walking over to her cousin she whispered to Lynn the code word, Pound Town, she knew it was Mr. Thaddeus Kofi from Vegas. Lynn knew the guy and informed Sunny of that.

"Girl, he is fine and plus girl he is my baby daddy cousin. What the heck is going on." She laughed to herself. "Guess I lost the bet huh? Have fun and call me or I'm calling the police." The two hugged as Sunny turned to Thaddeus. He escorted her to the exit door. The two of them had a little pep in their steps, almost a little trot out of the club, so happy to hear what was about to happen.

When Thaddeus hit the door of the club, he immediately powered walked to his truck, hitting the alarm so the truck would automatically start. Sunny was following close behind, following closely behind him was the woman who had been riding his dreams, thoughts, and mind for the last couple months since he left Vegas. So her name is Sunny. Thaddeus kept saying her name to himself in his mind until it became a song to his heart.

Sunny also was happy she found the man she longs for in her mind, heart and to feel him on her body again. Her name is Sunny.

Chapter 6

Her name is Sunny since Thaddeus thought of her as a ray of Sunshine to him. He was nervous as he arrived at his condo during what was a partially silent ride, but small talk. Thaddeus and Sunny kept taking glances at one another during the ride, the sexual tension was evident. He remembered that not much talking was done when they got to his hotel, which made him angry. Thaddeus wished he had asked some questions at least her name then, how could a woman hold his thoughts like she did.

With nervous hands he opened the door to his condo. He led Sunny inside only to turn to her and lock his lips onto hers. She welcomed his kiss without any hesitation or restraints. Their tongues began to dance with one another, matching each other's essence during their intimate kissing session. Love was in the air for the two of them.

Thaddeus was turned on by Sunny real bad, he thought those feelings had died deep down inside of him. What was it out of sight out of mind? It appears that she had some of the same feelings as well.

Sunny was about five six feet tall, with thick curves the curly coils she sported made her beautiful skin and amber eyes pop. This woman was flawless, as the maxi dress turned him on, especially the stilettos heels she wore. Thaddeus was taller than Sunny but the shoes brought her up to Thaddeus' chin. He loved a woman that was confident, and Sunny was all that.

Once inside the condo the two were at each other immediately, Thaddeus was filling up on Sunny as she welcomed every touch he delivered. He pulled her dress up over her head as to see her large full perky breast, they looked just as they did that night. He began to kiss her all over her face down into her chest. The slight moan that escaped her lips had turned Thaddeus on.

"Sunny, I've been thinking about you and that night for the last month," he told her. "When I didn't get your name or phone number I was mad at myself, especially after you didn't call."

It was silent as Thaddeus continued to kiss and fondle all over Sunny's body, he was tired of playing when he snatched her thongs down and relieved himself from his underwear. Her scent was so bold, and fresh Thaddues was about to erupt without being inside of Sunny. He asked, as he lead her toward the sofa,

"Come sit on my dick, I want to look into your eyes while you ride me." Sunny sat on top of Thaddeus as he slid her down on top of his hard erection. He was in paradise, Sunny rode him like her life depended on it. She reached back, fondling his balls as she bucked in a harmonic way. The moans that escaped Thaddeus' mouth made her bend down and hover her mouth on top of his. Thaddeus was in complete ecstasy; his mind was blown again. Sunny threw her head back and welcomed all of Thaddeus inside of her every inch. When she felt him almost about to explode she hopped off of him and closed her mouth over his tip to flick her tongue a few times. Thaddeus couldn't move; he was stuck.

"Sunny, wait ...." Thaddeus couldn't finish his sentence due to Sunny kissing him passionately as she bounced down on his dick clenching her muscles to bring his climax out of him. Thaddeus hollered like a girl, while holding onto Sunny's waist. climbed up onto him and tried to slide down onto his dick. The two of them had both enjoyed that moment and had to catch their breaths. Sunny was now laying on top of Thaddeus' chest as he had fallen over on the sofa. It was another twenty minutes before they had moved and Thaddeus brought in a cloth to clean her up.

"Let's do this the correct way," Thaddeus was looking at Sunny with a huge smile on his face. "Hello, my name is Thaddeus. It's nice to meet you." He began with his name then told her some things about him that weren't on the business card he left with her. "Oh so you threw it away huh?" Sunny was smiling up at Thaddeus when she spoke. He was smitten by her soft-spoken voice.

"Hi, Thaddeus it's nice meeting you. You're a handsome man I'm sure this isn't a first time for you to behave in this manner with a woman." She was being sarcastic. "My name is Sunny, I'm from the south. When we met I was at a seminar myself. I didn't throw your card away, there was so much going on with me." Sunny explained to him the past trauma and that she wasn't thinking she would ever see him again. What Sunny said to him was that she had called him but didn't leave a message she told him. "I tried twice but got too nervous to leave it."

The next couple hours they spent getting out the pleasantries and planned to see each other again. We must not leave out the fact that the intimacy wasn't left out, the two of them Thaddeus welcomed her to stay until the morning which she didn't turn him down since she was staying at a hotel currently.

"Good night, Sunny," Thaddeus showed her to his guest room giving her some privacy although they had just pounded each other's brains out.

"Good night Thaddeus, I truly enjoyed you." She said as she closed the door.

Thaddeus was lingering outside the door with his mind completely blown. He didn't think he would ever see her again; it surprised him that she was at his cousin's club with his girlfriend. The conversation would have been had if he knew her name. Thaddeus was sure that telling Nathan, his cousin the woman's name he wouldn't know, to tell Thaddeus that his girlfriend had a cousin named Sunny. The smile on his face was huge, as he thought to himself Oh we go together Sunny, real bad.

*****

"What's up Thaddeus," Sam called out as he went into his office suite. Today Thaddeus had an extra pep in his step as we thought of last night when he ran into Sunny, as it kept playing in his mind. He was so happy to finally place a name with the woman who rode his thoughts since the convention in Vegas.

"Hi, Sam what's up?" he replied with a smile plastered on his face. Thaddeus' smile was like he was auditioning for a commercial for a dentist commercial.

"So what's the word, you practically skipping up on her today. Who is she?" Sam knew something was different with her boss and she liked it on him.

"Well, you will see in due time, I've been doing so much lately that will change my life for the good." Thaddeus replied.

Getting back to work, Thaddeus was able to focus on his clients although he did slip up and went a little too far with the sensual sexual massage of his client Karen. He was thankful that she asked so he obliged and gave in.

The final client for the day Thaddeus has been extremely busy, he enjoyed giving his clients all they requested and needed from him. Continuing to reflect on the way he put his Brand to use gaining so many clients, his team was awesome.

"Welcome, is this your first time at the Majestic Massage Spa? In Magic, the head masseuse here. I see you have chosen our sensual hot oil massage.

Another day of pleasure at Majestic Massage Spa." He greeted the woman with a smile and advised her that he would be doing her massage and if she had any questions to please let him know.

"Thank you, I'm Regina and I'm excited, my husband gave this massage to me. So I'm sure you will give me something to report back." She started with a smile. Thaddeus returned the gesture as he walked her over to the table to pick out a choice of oils she liked. He advised her that the oil had a candle to accompany it also. She was intrigued by all the knowledge he had on the product. Thaddeus led her to the changing room after he took a glance again at the choice of massage she had paid for. It was one of his many favorites, the deep tissue, upper body with an intense vaginal play using exotic toys.

"You ready Ms. Regina? He asked her if she needed to relax as much as she could. She obliged once she felt his touch. It usually took about five minutes for the woman to truly unwind however Regina was ready and she enjoyed every bit of the massage. Thaddeus understood as he got further into the massage why her husband requested all the bells and whistles. Thinking to himself he was saying 'Damn she has climaxed several times just from him touching her non sensual hot spots, he must be lost with her." During his final round of pleasing her with the toys he asked her if she was all right.

"Magic, I'm telling you what has happened in this room has changed my life." Regina stated as she was in her final winddown moment. Thaddeus had given her some tips to take home with her.

"Your welcome Ms. Regina, and I've already sent the order for your oils and candles to the front desk. I'm sure your husband will enjoy them." Thaddeus gave her a handshake as he escorted her to the font to check out with Sam.

Today has been fast tracked, extremely busy at the Majestic Massage Spa. Thaddeus was tidying up his loose ends. His mind drifted to thinking of Sunny, having spent another night with her and learning who she is placed a permanent smile on his face. The future was looking bright, his pockets were growing from being a successful business owner. In his last vision board he placed a new location where the clientele could be more exotic to the culture of sensual massages. The brand would have to be developed to get the word out.

Heading home Thaddeus decided to send his new woman a text but headed to Melissa's house instead of going straight home. It was something he would soon have to stop. Thaddeus knew that hurt people; hurt people he didn't want to get that kind of label on his name.

Once Thaddeus was outside of Melissa's house he sat there for about an hour until he went to the door.

"Hey, come in." Melissa told him, looking at him. There were no words spoken. Melissa just did what she would always satisfy him on his command. Something wasn't right with Thaddeus; it wasn't his usual request of her; he only wanted her to just give him some head and then he left.

"Take care, Melissa, I'll call you sometime soon."

The ride home Thaddeus felt so guilty for being with another woman when he knew his heart would soon belong to Sunny.

Chapter 7

The last few days went off well. It was routine for Thaddeus at Majestic. Each client that came into the establishment was generous with their tipping for the staff. It was all paying off for Thaddeus, however he was still feeling empty inside. He made a mental note to contact Sunny later on to get her to come over. Although she explained to him she wasn't looking for anything serious he had already fallen for her. It was during the conversations they had on their career path and goals. Thaddeus noticed how intrigued she seemed in what he did for a living. While he showed her some of his line of work she responded with respect for him since it was his choice of career.

"So you do the majority of sensual massages or just the regular." Sunny asked.

"I tend to do more healing massages than personal injuries. The preference would be for me to do more natural healing techniques." He explained while she expressed with passion in his voice.

Sunny told him about her work as well. He was extremely interested and then proceeded to tell her that he wouldn't mind getting to know her more. IT was everything in her to tell him no but she was smitten by his strong voice, handsome looks, and sensitive touch.

"Thaddeus, come look at this for a second," Sam the office manager called out to him. He had been on a brief break from work and he was daydreaming in his office.

"Sure, Sam, give me about five minutes and I'll be right over." He replied.

The numbers that Sam owed him was impressive, in the last three months business was booming for them. They had full calendars for each one of the masseuses working in the building. Rodney and Charlie were doing well, Thaddeus liked that fact Charlie had most of the sensual massages on her schedule with both men and women. He loved her professionalism.

"Thanks, Sam, he believes his clients may be upset when I cancel all my sensual massages. The time may be near for me to let it go." Thaddeus was contemplating letting that part of his career go since he was looking to settle down in the near future. That was something he had talked about with his cousin but not totally with his partners. "Sure boss," Sam said with a smile. "Let me get on that and I'll get you your dates and time. Just me being on my job, does that young lady that you have glued to your phone have something to do with that decision?"

The smile that Thaddeus had on his face said all that needed to be said. There wasn't any need for words. Sam just smiled back, going to her laptop to complete her given task.

It was late afternoon when one of Thaddeus clients came into the office. He escorted her back to his room.

"Hello Karen, it's been a while how are you?" she responded with a smile then she asked could they get started.

"Yes, no problem," scanning the fact sheets, Thaddeus noticed that she was too distant. He began the session with Karen, he is always professional so he continued on. The next thirty minutes was totally geared to Karen as Thaddeus finished up. "Okay Karen, we are complete."

"Thank you Magic, I wanted to tell you this has been such a pleasure. You have helped me so much in areas that I was concerned about sexually." Karen was letting Thaddeus know she was having problems so with her coming to the massages got her to relax and be aware of her desires.

"You're so welcome, so glad this was able to help you. He wanted to let you know that your referrals have been great. So If you are ever in need of further assistance I'd be glad to help you." Thaddeus walked her out as he thanked her again.

Thaddeus was finished up his day to head home when he received a tax from Melissa. While he wasn't in the mood for her he went ahead and swung by her place. Since he had met Sunny, Thaddeus wasn't feeling too much for her, the sex wasn't as great anymore he was in need of more than a temporary sexual pleasure.

Melissa: Can you stop over , I'm at my shop.
Thaddeus: Yes, be by in twenty minutes.

Pulling into the parking lot of Melissa salon Thaddeus thought of the woman he saw leaving out of the parking lot in a white, Ford Explorer. He turned around to assure he wasn't seeing things.

Thaddeus called Melissa to come let him in since he couldn't access entry from the door. He saw the reflection of a person walking to the door.

"Come in," Melissa extended as she opened the door. "You look handsome baby," she said to Thaddeus as he gave her a look. The way her hair was distressed on her head she had tears in her eyes.

"What's up? Why did you get tears in your eyes?" he noticed them asking her what the reason for her distraught look was.

Melissa explained that her new designer she chose had pulled a muscle after being asked to help her move. "She was cool with it but it appears, we both hadn't realized the heaviness of the table." She was sniffling. "I let go some and it caused her to drop it too and fall. She's probably going to sue me, why couldn't I have waited?" Melissa was now in a full-blown cry.

"Look, hopefully she didn't hurt herself really badly. You shouldn't have asked her but I get it that independent woman bullshit you be on." He was now looking at Melissa with sympathetic eyes, pulling her into his embrace. Thaddeus asked to look around at the completion of the design. The details of the decorations showed that it was prepared exclusively for Missy. He noticed how the colors she chose gave a relaxation vibe for her clients. "So this person was very thorough with the design and placing of the decorations. I really like it Missy." She blushed from him using her nickname. Thaddeus hoped he wasn't putting any wrong thoughts into her head about them; it was just a sexual relationship only. He had to express that to her several times but the small things he saw her doing was leading to her probably stepping out of line. Melissa led him back into her office and as he went back a familiar scent hit his nose he knew all too well. It was that

"Thank you, I did give her your company card for a massage if she needed it." His eyes turned and locked with Melissa. Thaddeus knew exactly who it was once she gave the name of the business. The woman of his dreams, and who held his heart.

They talked for another few minutes when Thaddeus couldn't resist himself. He instructed Melissa to, "Lean over the desk. Press your face to the top of it. Hold onto the far edge with both your hands." Melissa complied but turned her head so she could see what he was doing. Thaddeus' words were somewhat demonic, she thought, but she did follow his instructions.

Melissa felt Thaddeus run his hand over her ass. "Nice firm and round. I like this view on you." He slipped his hand lower down onto her calf and slowly ran his hand up the inside of her leg just as high as the top of her leggings. She felt her calves tremble at the touch of his hands on her body. Thaddeus knew he was good at what he did as he continued to run his hands up and down her stockings. During this he drifted into a head space that he only smelled the scent of another woman he knew was inside the shop. Thaddeus then asked Melissa, "What's the persons or company that you used for decorating?" he managed to get that out in a normal tone unlike his demands of her instructions being spread out on top of her five thousand-dollar desk.

"What? Why are you asking about another woman when I'm here." She asked, as she tried to turn her head to see what Thaddeus was doing. He eased his semi erect penis out to rub on her leggings to give her assurance she was about to get the dick. "It's new called Sensational Designs or something like that." Melissa answered.

"Not asking about any one in particular, you did refer to her.

That did it for Thaddeus. He applied pressure to Melissa's inner thighs and he ripped her leggings to see her center. The ripping of the foil was music to Melissa ears while she loved how he delivered the much-needed strokes of pleasure it was not what she expected.

Thadeus was in a zone, he entered Melissa with so much force as leaned back thinking of Sunny. When he had felt himself almost about to explode he removed himself from Melissa turning her to face him, telling her to open her mouth. "Open up so I can feel those lips and warm mouth." She complained it was like anything for him. With about three forceful thrust Thaddeus began to go in on Melissa's throat. It was like he totally forgot he was in her mouth. Thaddeus felt himself about to release when he pulled back on her long weave making her almost gag while he released himself inside of her. "Damn, that was amazing."

When Thaddeus came from the bathroom inside of Melissa's office, he handed her a towel to wipe her mouth. The tears that were on her face, he ignored them. Melissa wasn't going to change it by saying anything as she did the last time they had been intimate. She knew her place but of course she wanted more, most women did. Thaddeus was a great catch, any woman would be happy to be with him, or even seen in public with him.

"You good? Did you hurt yourself?" He was asking Melissa to show he does have a heart. Just as he was speaking to her his phone was buzzing in his pocket because he had an incoming message.

"No, but thanks for asking. I want to know if you can be my plus one at the Fashion Expo Ball?" Melissa was taking a chance on asking knowing the relationship was nonexistent.

"Let me be clear Melissa, you know what it is with us. That would sure to confuse you or anyone else. I'm good at that." He let her down then proceeded to leave so the conversation wouldn't go wrong.

Melissa walked Thaddeus to the door with him laying a kiss on her forehead.

Hoping in his Range Rover, Thaddeus jumped in heading home to relax after a successful day at work. Him being with Melissa was a bonus to relieve some extra stress. Bumping his summer jams playlist he noticed the vibration of his phone again. Pulling it out to check he saw it was a few text messages sent. The first three were from Sam at the shop then Nathan, his cousin, the final two were from Sunny. His eyes lit up as well as the memory of her scent.

Sunny: Hi, I had an incident where I needed company at the ER.
Sunny: The Central General Hospital if you aren't busy. Your name is at the reception desk.

Reading Sunny's text messages over for the tenth time, Thaddeus heads to Central General to see about his woman. Although they hadn't made any official titles on what they where he claimed her as his.

When he pulled up to the ER parking the attendant showed him the parking garage and entrance.

Sitting in the waiting area until the nurse came over had Thaddeus on edge, he didn't know what to expect. The brief description of the incident explained by Melissa was minor, but the whole ER visit was serious. The nurse was walking over towards Thaddeus, "Mr. Kofi? Mrs. Stallings is this way, follow me sir." The nurse escorted him to the back when he saw Sunny he was instantly upset. She had a temporary sling on her arm.

"Hi Beautiful Sunshine, are you okay." Thaddeus walked over towards Sunny reaching out for her.

"Yes, I'm better now with the pain meds and temporary sling for my shoulder.," Sunny explained to him what happened to cause her to end up in the ER. "It was horrible. I knew I should have said no."

"Well, it was a learning experience, I'm glad you had come in to be seen. "Thaddeus sat with Sunny while the nurse gave the doctor her final instructions. The nurse had her sign the paperwork, after having me sign a consent to assure she gets home sage. She couldn't drive due to the medication that they gave her for pain.

It's in the north end of the emergency department, you can bring it to my house. Yes my house, come on now I wouldn't have said it if I didn't mean it Miles. Thanks again I'll make sure you are straight. Thaddeus was telling his regular mechanic to bring Sunny's car to his home so she can have it when she is able to drive.

"Thaddeus you could have towed my car to my condo. How am I going to get around without a car?" Sunny was trying to plead her case; he wasn't hearing anything on which she was speaking.

"Stop, Sunny, I've made the final decision regarding your care and safety for the next forty-eight hours." He continued walking while the patient attendant came to retrieve her. Thaddeus let them both know he would go get the car.

Sunny gave Thaddeus her prescriptions to pick up from the Walgreen from her home, although he wasn't dropping her off at home. He did allow her to go in while they grabbed her toiletries. Thaddeus was assuring that she grabbed what was needed to stay for a few days.

"Is that all you need?" he was looking at the large overnight bag Sunny had. "You got enough for a few weeks don't you? Let me find out you are moving in with me." They both laughed as they walked out of Sunny's condo.

"Real funny," she protested while letting him know it had her favorites inside. The drive was thirty minutes from Sonny's place. She drifted off to sleep just as they pulled off with her prescriptions.

Thaddeus carried a sleeping Sunny into his house, taking her to the guest room on the bottom floor. It was tempting for him to take her to his master suite but didn't want to totally overstep any unspoken boundaries they hadn't yet discussed.

Kissing her forehead he allowed her to sleep as he went off to his room.

Tonight was long as Thaddeus had some serious thinking to do. He had already said to himself that he wanted to make some changes and after being with Melissa he knew that he had to cut that off. How he was going to pursue Sunny wholeheartedly. When he saw her at the ER, banned up scared him, especially knowing that she was injured at his own off again girl. Thaddeus has to come clean or things just may blow up in his face. Leaving Sunny in his guest room was hard for him knowing he wanted to go be with her bad. First he remembered he had to wash off the remnants of him and Melissa's sexual session.

Once Thaddeus finished his shower he prayed to allow his words to come out correct so he can properly claim his woman who was just down the hall in his home.

Chapter 8

Melissa was waking up from a night of one-to-many margaritas. She was thinking of how embarrassed she felt to have been played by Thaddeus. Although she did recall on several occasions during the situation-ship he explained nothing would come of it. Melissa couldn't understand why since they did what couples do some of the time. Thaddeus was a great catch and she was upset that he didn't want her like she wanted him now after all these years.

In Melissa's mind she was having a full conversation with herself; he thought this a joke. *I'm going down to that little spa and claiming my man. Let him know how much I love him.*

With an oversize black T-shirt, her skinny jeans, and her black Air Max she was ready. Pulling her nice three sixty lace front wig up in a ponytail Melissa was one way to Majestic Massage Spa to stake her claim for her man. It was humiliating, and embarrassing to her to be passed over in public like she was. Melissa had told a few of her close friends that Thaddeus and her were exclusive only to see him pushing up on another woman in front of her.

In Melissa's head she had already planned to walk in the shop and demand Thaddeus see her and make the commitment that she wanted. She was livid just thinking of how she had played herself.

When Melissa got to the Spa the parking lot wasn't full; she was looking for her Thaddeus truck then saw it parked in the far corner of the parking lot. Melissa walked to the door pulling it open eyeing the area. In her mind she was about to cut up Thaddeus, but didn't see him when she walked in.

"Hi, Melissa what's up," Sam greeted Melissa with a smile. Sam could see that Melissa was looking really delusional.

"I know Thaddeus is here, get him out here," Melissa began to talk loud towards Sam. "He thinks he can just treat me any kind of way like my feelings don't matter."

"Just a minute Melissa, why don't you sit down until I call him up front." Sam stated

Just as they both had a moment of silence Melissa jumped up and grabbed a small statue off the table and threw it up to make a statement. Sam turned looking over her shoulder at Melissa.

"Hey, calm down, I'm going have to make you leave." Sam rolled her eyes as she went to get Thaddeus.

Sam came towards Thaddeus and his co-workers with a deranged look on her face.

"Thaddeus, I'm going to say this once. Your THOT of a girl or client is out front making a whole scene. She is loud, embarrassing herself regarding an appointment that we both know she doesn't have." Sam continued to express the way Melissa was acting in front of clients that caused one lady to leave.

"Hold on Sam, did you call the police? It sounds like it may have escalated beyond my control. Melissa knows that she isn't allowed here anymore." Thaddeus had to result in banning her due to last week's antics. He didn't escort her to the ball then she saw him with Sunny in the market and lost her mind. Needless to say he had already slept with Melissa a few more times after that. One of the many reasons he stopped her from coming to the shop and pursuing him was when they had been out at happy hour. Melissa had pretended to be extremely drunk that she needed an escort home. Thaddeus didn't want her to go home alone so he took her. Big mistake she managed to drug him and they woke up naked with the appearance of having unprotected sex. Thaddeus was livid; he jumped into action knowing that he needed to act fast so he contacted Sam, to get the cocktail recipe to prevent a pregnancy after unprotected sex. To his relief Sam came over to her place dropping off a bag. It was to look like he was getting a change of clothes but it was more. Thaddeus cooked breakfast for Melissa feeding her the Plan B pill so she wouldn't end up pregnant, he wasn't going to be trapped into a permanent relationship with a woman he wasn't into. That alone was another strike against Melissa. Now here she was trying to persuade Thaddeus she was the one, but no she wasn't doing these kinds of toxic antics.

"Yes, I called them, they are on the way. She told me to go to hell and fuck the police. Thaddeus this isn't right she is rude, and ugly." Sam was correct while Charlie told them she would handle the craziness that was going on.

"No, I'll go out and talk to her since she wants to be seen by me." Thaddeus walked towards the lobby when the police also arrived. The two officers that entered were glad to discuss the outcome if Melissa didn't come to her senses and leave. It was just so that one of the offices was a frequent client of Rodney's;

she enjoyed the massages after a long week at work, as the other officer just looked around.

Once Melissa realized she was about to go to jail, but not until she tried to expose Thaddeus for doing his job. "You up in here giving happy endings, slinging your dick, to all your clients. When you can have me, what we share is more than just sex, you are just fighting it." Melissa was displaying anger and bitterness from being rejected. During her fiasco of a throwing fit. She had managed to tear up the lobby area. Melissa looked around at her handy work. The statues she threw one had almost hit one of the waiting clients, they moved quickly to avoid the raft of the women who were hollering and screaming. Melissa had thrown magazines on the floor, broken up the candles in the display. Her handy work was horrible. The few clients inside the office had already been checked in and signed the NDA so no video of the scene Melissa made was going to go any further than that office.

Finally once the officers got her calm no charges were filed against her but a warning if she returns she would be arrested. It wasn't no more than half a second before the officer walked out of the property that Melissa was being persuaded for bad language and obstruction of property, one of the clients in the office was bleeding from some glass that had broken in the raft by Melissa. This would teach her a lesson, as he looked on to see the reaction that she may get from Thaddeus for her behavior.

Chapter 9

Sam, Rodney, and Charlie came to Thaddeus office once the situation of Melissa died down. Everyone was looking over at Thaddeus for an explanation.

"Spill it Magic," Charlie said with a smirk on her face.

"Yes, Mr. Long Stroke, with these happy endings you passing out," Rodney couldn't control his laughter, looking at his best friend. The way he demonstrated the long stroke was hilarious.

Thaddeus tried to ignore the antics but he himself burst out laughing at the comments his friends had made regarding the show that Melissa put on. Soon as the laughter died down, Thaddeus went on to explain what drove or would make Melissa act up on him. "See I knew she would eventually try to expect more than what it was explained to her we had." Thaddeus was telling his friends that he told her it was over, done that he wouldn't be giving out any more of his magic stick. She went in on him, especially when he couldn't escort her to the event. "You know when I showed up with Sunny, she tried to curve her at the event."

"So you telling me that she asked you to be her plus one, you declined and showed up with your new bae? Oh heck no I know it was a drama." Sam asked as they waited on Thaddeus to give the specifics.

"Y'all know that I've been going through my own personal battles. When I met Sunny it hit my heart differently and I know she was sent to me and I acted on it after I found out she was living here locally." Thaddeus signed as he continued on telling his team that he knew it was actually live at first sight. "She is the one."

"I see, was it on the trip? "Rodney asked, "You had seemed distant on the flight back so I take it to be you was lovesick."

"Yes, that shit is real." Thaddeus stated. In his explanation he proceeded letting them know he was going to do anymore triple x addition to the sensual massages nor the vaginal tantra massages. Thaddeus told Charlie she could have his clients if Rodney couldn't fit them in. Clearing up all loose ends on the job the three carried on with their day.

Thaddeus saw his schedule for the rest of the week he was pleased but it showed that he had one sensual massage on his calendar.

"Sam, come into my office please." Thaddeus called out to her over the intercom phone system. Once she was inside his office she knew what he was going to ask before he got out the words.

"Yes, I know it's from our new boo, she made the appointment over a week ago on the online calendar. When I noticed her name I left it for you." Sam had a huge smile plastered on her face. "Boss man, you're going to have to really show her what you do to earn all the big bucks, Magic." Laughing Sam left out of Thaddeus office within also in deep laughter.

The night was fast approaching an end when Thaddeus received a message from Sunny to come over. He immediately responded to her text with a time he thought he would be arriving.

Sunny: Hi, can you come over tonight?

Thaddeus: Yes sweetheart around 8:30 (smiley emoji)

Thaddeus was sitting in his truck when he felt his notifications going off again. In his gut he had a feeling it was something that would be off. Checking it was a few text messages from Melissa. She was going in on him again on his betrayal, threatening him to tell his new girl the truth. One text message stood out the most was her stating, "I'll show her a receipt that we shared more than a simple relationship. Receipts of the same night you were with me the same night as her." Thaddeus had a knot in his throat not realizing that he didn't share the whole truth with Sunny about his prior relationship. With the woman who was mean mugging her at the fashion gala that night.

"Come in," Sunny was holding the door open for Thaddeus. He was happy to see her beautiful smile when the both leaned into one another for an embrace with a passionate kiss. Gathering each other's breath, Sunny sat on the sofa with Thaddeus. She began to speak about a message from a woman regarding him. It was very vague in the questions that were asked about her and Thaddeus when he asked Sunny, "Baby, show me the message please." She obliged; It wasn't a photo of a person but of a space he was familiar with. When he saw it he immediately knew who it was, Melissa.

When Thaddeus broke it down to Sunny she wasn't in the bit of upset regarding his relationship with Melissa but to find out who she was made it awkward. "Sunny, when we met I was broken in so many ways, the fact that we both had issues of which we wasn't sure. I'd thought I wouldn't see you ever again but hoped that we could get together again. It was love at first site with you, for me to withhold any information regarding another woman I apologize." Thaddeus was pouring out his heart again. "Sunny I love you and want to spend these months getting to know you." Grabbing her into his arms he landed a passionate kiss to her lips. She welcomed his tongue into her mouth as their hands began fondling each other. Their kissing led to Sunny taking the loop off of Thaddues pants to expose him as she went to work fondling his semi erection. He moaned in her mouth, as he fell into sync with her movements. Sunny pushed him back into the sofa where he fell with his head hanging over the back of the chair. With Sunny going down on Thaddeus he was enjoying it so much but not as much as Sunny was. She began to pleasure him as she did each time, her skills was five stars better than what was seen on Porn Hub or any other triple x sites.

"Baby, yesssss that feels so..." was all that he got out before he grabbed onto Sunny's head. She took all of him down her throat using her tonsils with her mouth muscles to bring him to total pleasure. Thaddeus began to swell in her mouth and he released all his seeds down Sunny's throat. He couldn't do anything but lay back to gather his breath. Sunny laid with him for a few minutes just to allow them to both enjoy one another.

The two had drifted off to sleep only for Thaddeus to wake Sunny up down between her legs. He had been down savoring the flavor of her scent as he brought her to a few organisms. Sunny's eyes flew open as she arched her back pressing her honey pot into Thaddeus' mouth. He used his fingers to assist in bringing her another orgasm. When Sunny woke completely up she wrapped her hands around Thaddeus head, she pulled him in her as her legs began to shake to another orgasm. "Oh, baby that feels so good, yes keep going I'm almost," as she moaned out Thaddeus name. Raising up Thaddeus pulled back and eased himself into her opening. The way they both began to grind into one another was more than enough for each other. "Yes baby, you feel so good." Both of them said in unison.

"Sunny, I love you." Thaddeus professed his love for her during this intimate moment. He became so caught up when it was time to release himself nothing mattered but for him to be one with her. Sunny smiled hearing Thaddeus' confession as she kissed him.

"I love you too," she stated.

"Sunny, I'm about to cum baby." Just as he said that he release deep inside her walls. Laying deep into his arms Sunny kissed Thaddeus passionately. She told him that she had something to share with him. Getting up to go get a towel to clean him up, she first took care of herself.

"Here baby, come into the bedroom." Sunny instructed him. Walking behind her Thaddeus popped her on the behind.

Inside her bedroom, Sunny went over to her purse to retrieve something. She was walking with less pep in her step as she came over where he was standing. Once she got to him, he saw the tears that had formed in her eyes, "Hey, what's wrong, we shared a great moment baby. Why are you looking that way."

Sunny was nervous, she just came right out with it, looking into his eyes. "I'm pregnant Thaddeus." One lone tear fell down her face. He pulled her into his arms, using his thumb to wipe her tears away. "I know it's not what we planned. I took a home test but when I went to get my physical, they told me." Sunny was crying tears now." Thaddeus hadn't stated anything yet to assure her of what he thought.

"Baby don't cry. It's alright I'm not upset. We will be fine." Thaddeus gave Sunny some assurance that he wasn't going to run out on her. They both knew the relationship was fresh, but each time no protection was used.

Once Thaddeus made sure that Sunny was fine he prepared to leave. He went to leave when she asked him if he was sure about the news, "Are you okay?" he told her eyes as she walked him out the door. Giving Sunny a kiss on her lips he left heading home.

Chapter 10

"Melissa Freeman, you made bail," the bailiff called out to Melissa. When she realized that her sneakiness backfired on her she was upset. Prior to her drugging Thaddeus drank one night after he told her he was moving on and she was done. They had unprotected sex multiple times in hopes that she would become pregnant to keep Thaddeus in her life. While it worked but she didn't know he knew something was right. Thinking back on that date she was upset because somehow after a few weeks later she was bent over in her bathroom with severe cramps. She was having a miscarriage, how was that happening Melissa was upset that led her to show up at Thaddeus job. Then she showed up at Sunny's place of business, to try and expose the relationship between her and Thaddeus. To her knowledge she thought he was just like most men, leaving her after he had gotten what he wanted. Melissa didn't have many friends, so she wasn't sure who had bailed her out of jail for showing up at Sunny's place of business. When she came out of jail she saw someone, to her surprise Sam, Thaddeus' receptionist. "Come on don't look like that, you best thank the heavens because I would have left your crazy ass here to rot."

"Why did he?" Melissa was asking Sam why did Thaddeus bail her out.

"He knew your crazy self-had no money like this to get out, nor did you know a bondsman." Sam barked, "Come on, let's get out of here before someone sees me."

Melissa was grateful, but still hurt when she was explaining to Sam what happened. Little did Melissa know the Plan B cocktail that she was given was made by Sam. When Thaddeus called Sam he knew that the damage was done sleeping with Melissa unprotected was not ever in his plan. Sam told her to get her life together, to apologize to Sunny and she may ask them to drop all charges against her.

Although what Sam was saying made so much logical sense Melissa was too stubborn to comply with the request. It was in Melissa's mind that Thaddeus belonged to her and she to him. The times when they had been intimate he always told her that it was only sex nothing more or less. When she drugged him she thought he was more into her but it was the drugs she added to his drink. Melissa knew all too well that she would never be the main girl for him.

The circles they were in were different and then to add fuel to the fire, she couldn't stay in her lane.

"Do you hear me Melissa," Sam asked her, only for her to stare off into the air. Melissa's mind was going a mile a minute. First for her to even be in jail behind a man whom she couldn't have. Then for her to damage his property and his woman's property. The woman he made known that he was going to be with and not her.

"Hump, I'm not doing that, she got my man and I want him back. I love him, Sam." Melissa confessed to Sam .

"Girl, give it up, he has healed and moved on. You are going to have to stop looking bad. Listen, put on your big girl panties, and move around. It shouldn't be hard for you to find your own man." Sam told her with a mothering look on her face. Melissa wasn't trying to hear her but she did nod in agreement.

Melissa was home resting when she strolled through her social media accounts. When she came onto Sunny's page she only saw how her business and a few of her personal photos looked. It wasn't but a few that she saw to see Sunny was pregnant and that Thaddeus was in some of the photos. Nothing else was showing of the two flaunting their relationship in her face. Melissa became livid until she thought of her conversation with Sam.

It was after Melissa went over to Thaddeus page that she saw him hugged up with Sunny on a lounge chair. The two of them were looking into one another's eyes. The photo looked like it was older than today's date but it still made Melissa upset. Her thoughts were just running wild. How could he be so cruel, she would say. How could I not be good enough for him? Why did I allow myself to love him? After another thirty minutes she poured herself a drink, when the pain hit her in her stomach. When Melissa made it to the restroom, her body was aching and then she saw all the blood running down her legs. She knew what was happening, the big secret she was trying to hide was no longer. Falling down on the floor Melissa cried as she knew then it was all over any chance of trying to get Thaddeus to remain in her life.

"I will not be out done," Melissa said as she began to get herself together. She took a shower and mended herself up enough to allow the miscarriage take its place. "Before this is over Thaddeus will not ignore me."

Melissa laid on the sofa until she fell off to sleep.

Chapter 11

"What's up cousin, I hadn't heard from you in a few days, How is my lil cousin?" Lynn had called to check on Sunny, she was with her when she found out about the baby. It came as a surprise to Sunny when she found herself leaning over the toilet one morning before going to one of her clients.

"Girl it's horrible, why didn't you say anything about this when you were pregnant with Natalie? I would have been prepared at least." Sunny was asking since it was all of a sudden for her. The way the morning sickness just showed up was a shock to her.

Lynn talked to Sunny about the ends and outs of being pregnant, and what to expect. She told her that no one could predict what kind of craving or weight gain or loss that a person would experience. Lynn advised Sunny to try to keep all stress to a minimum. What she said next was what Sunny wants to hear.

"Sunny the sex has to continue," she said, "What kept me calm and eased some of the changes that went unnoticed was the attention I got during the pregnancy from Natalie's dad." Lynn telling Sunny those things gave her some relief. Sunny knew her and Thaddeus' sexual relationship was priceless. It hadn't gotten dead; it was full of love and excitement.

"Lynn you are a crazy girl, I know we will be doing plenty of that. You know I even went to the sugar and salt place to make us some signature body scrubs." Sunny was telling Lynn how she was making all her dreams come true with Thaddeus giving him ideas to explore on her as she did the exact same with him. Thaddues loved how Sunny was into the thoughts of fulfilling her fantasies. His sex drive was over the top.

The relationship that Sunny and Thaddeus started out was only for a one night of sexual pleasure now over the last few months it's become a plus one. When Thaddeus expressed himself to her she wasn't sure that she wanted to be in a relationship; it was just to be one night in the sinful city of Vegas. While Sunny truly enjoyed every moment of it she was even more happy to find him in the same town as she relocated. Her mind drifted to her pain to the current pleasure she is experiencing. The new relationship and now a new life that will be approaching the world in the next five months. It was one night of passion that led to a lifetime of commitment. Sunny wasn't feeling guilty when she thought of all the intimate trips she fulfilled with Thaddeus. In her mind it was a new addition that was made in fun, love, and excitement. Sunny was thinking back over things when she heard her name being called.

"Sunny, Sunny what are you doing girl, why haven't you answered me." Lynn asked, "You are not enough months to be experiencing brain fog, or delirious moments." She rolled her eyes at Lynn watching her laugh at her own antics.

"Sunny, seriously how are you feeling? Do you need anything?" Lynn continued asking about her health and if she had any craving. Then also she wanted to know about her and Thaddeus.

"Cousin, he is wonderful. That one-night stand was the best ever. We still have a few kinks in the relationship but overall it's wonderful." Sunny stated. "Next week we may be able to find out the sex of the baby. I'm happy that I won't be alone during this journey. He has been involved in everything, baby." Sunny explained. Then she got quiet on the phone, thinking of the scene with Melissa and Thaddeus. When they were at the ball, Sunny remembered that she was all in Thaddeus' face, when they thought she wasn't watching. He came to the event alone but once he saw her, Thaddeus was all over Sunny. She had that sling which she wore with her beautiful cocktail stress and some sandals that string up her legs. When Thaddeus noticed that another guy, Raymond, was checking for her he got heated. Although the Art District wasn't big she knew who Raymond was and so did Thaddeus.

"Hey Sunny, can I get you to have a drink with me." He asked her when Thaddeus was talking with Melissa. She told me I'm yes unaware that the insults from Melissa would be directed to her.

"Sure Raymond" she told him only for the moment to be cut short by Thaddeus coming to claim his woman. That evening Sunny left with Thaddeus and the rest of the night was of him telling her everything. The way they made love that night without protection could have just been the final bake of the baby in her belly. Sunny wasn't sure however she did remember multiple times no protection was used.

That afternoon Sunny was sitting in her office when she heard her door chime that someone had entered. Since she came into her office twice a week she hired a receptionist to be out front in case someone came in. Sunny continued with her work as normal until she heard the voices out front get louder than usual. Ear hustling wasn't her strongest point so she went to find out the big commotion. To her surprise was Melissa, being rude and very ugly towards her receptionist Beverly. Sunny didn't want to prolong the agonizing, ill treatment towards her worker.

"Excuse me, how can I help you?" she asked Melissa. The look of hate and disgust was all over her face. Sunny didn't know what to expect from her so she stood in enough distance from her. When Melissa tried to walk over towards her Sunny stated again, "How can I help you Missy?" That was the name that she knew her by from the contract work she did for her months ago. Now that she knew who Sunny was, she didn't want to take any chances in trying to attack her behind Thaddeus.

"Yes, you can help me. I wanted to let you know that we will have to share our man," she then started to rub on her belly trying to indicate that she was possibly pregnant. "You see I'm carrying Thaddeus' baby so we will be sharing him."

Sunny just looked at her with no kind of emotion, she then walked over to Beverly. When she did that Melissa tried to reach out towards her but missed and fell on to the floor. The sound of her fall was extremely loud, she was showing that she was in pain. Sunny asked Beverly to call the ambulance to get assistance to Melissa. The three ladies sat waiting for the ambulance to arrive when Sunny called Thaddeus to tell him what had happened. Once the EMT arrived they assisted Melissa on the gurney when she shouted I 'm going to sue you for injury as she bent over as if she was in pain.

"You attempted to assault Ms. Sunny; you can't sue anyone should sue it should be us." Beverly shouted towards Melissa.

"Try all you want, we have surveillance cameras that record inside and out," Sunny barked back at Melissa.

Thaddeus had arrived after all the commotion had passed; he was concerned about Sunny since she was actually the one who was carrying his child. The antics that Melissa told Sunny he had no recollection of that information at all. He assured Sunny that he would be getting to the bottom of whatever games that she was playing. Sunny's assistant told Thaddeus what happened as well then she left the office for the day.

"Bev, thank you so much you can take off the next week with pay. I believe I'm going to be working from home for a while, my calendar isn't too full." Sunny told her receptionist, who thanked her and walked out to her car.

Thaddeus helped Sunny pack up her bags and escorted her to her car. He was concerned that she may have been overexerted from all the activity with Melissa. Too much stress wasn't good for anyone, and he didn't want to have her stressed out behind another woman in which he wasn't interested.

"I placed all your bags in my car, ride with me I'll have someone bring your car to my house." Thaddeus was directing Sunny to his car, as he continued to apologize to her for the behavior of Melissa.

Sunny didn't fight the feeling she just went on without a fight. When she was seated in Thaddeus' truck she leaned over to open his door for him. He thanked her for the gesture with a long passionate kiss, "I have something for you when we get to my house," the smile he had on his face was huge. Sunny just smiled big thinking of what was in store for her when they arrived at his home.

"Wake up baby," Thaddeus had arrived at his place. "Sunny wake up," he had to tap on her shoulder, she had fallen asleep during the ride. Although Sunny was only in her second trimester she was extremely tired a lot. The doctor told her that her iron was low, but she wasn't sure of what she could do to keep her iron levels up.

"I'm up baby," Sunny responded, she placed her hand into Thaddeus to be helped into the house. Sunny immediately went over to the sofa to rest; she wasn't aware just how tired she was until mid-way into the ride.

Thaddeus had made her a cup of tea to help her relax then he placed some candles around the house to help soothe the moment. The scent was Sunny's favorite; he lit up the Black Love with a hint of sage and amber. Some music started playing in the background, as the lights began to dim down. Thaddues wasn't playing, he pulled out all the stops to help Sunny to relax. She enjoyed a moment like this with him, knowing that the next thing would be a massage that was long overdue. Looking over towards her man she saw him coming with a robe.

"Thaddeus you don't have to....," the passionate kiss he gave her melted the clothes she was wearing off of her body. Slipping into the robe she eased her body up against his firm muscles that she loved being next too. His biceps were huge as he helped her down onto the sofa. Thaddeus motioned for Sunny to give him her feet, which was his starting place today. While she threw her head back onto the sofa to relax as Thaddeus went in on her feet.

BUZZ, BUZZ was the sound that they both heard, it was familiar to Thaddeus. "What is that?" Sunny asked.

"Just relax, it's the oil that I'm going to use, it's is warm enough for me to apply now." The smile on her face made Thaddeus put a little pep in his step walking over to the warming pot. He poured some of the oil into his palms to apply to her feet as he worked it in deeply pressing on the points that helped her relax. When she hurt herself prior, Thaddeus told her how some places in her foot were essential to healing. He worked out some other kinks in her foot that were hurting when she walked. When he finished her feet he went up to her calve muscle all the way into her thighs. The sensation that came from the massage was putting Sunny to sleep. She was genuinely enjoying it, taking her mind off of the circus of events that happened early at her office.

Thirty minutes later Sunny was in a full snoring state, Thaddeus rendered a marvelous job of getting her to relax. He was worried about her and his unborn child. When Sunny called him to tell him what happened he dropped what he was doing to come to her aid. Telling his team that he wouldn't return for the day, he knew that she needed him. Thaddeus had called to check in once he took Sunny up to his bed placing her under the covers for her to fully rest.

Moving around Sunny realized she wasn't in her own bed; her mind was going back to the last few hours. She knew that Melissa had come to her job and Thaddeus came in to get her. The smell of something made Sunny's stomach churn, she was having an episode of that morning sickness. She got up and ran to the bathroom to spill her guts.

"Thaddeus," she called out to him to see if he could come in and help her. "Thaddeus can you come here, please." Leaning over into the toilet Sunny sat down in front of the toilet.

"Hey beautiful are you all right? What can I get you? Aww baby..." Thaddeus kneeled down to rub on her back as she continued to spill her guts in the toilet. This was new to the both of them. Once Sunny had completed her bout with the toilet she told Thaddeus she wanted to eat.

"I'm starving baby," sure sweetheart he replied as they headed down to the kitchen. Thaddeus was taking care of Sunny since he felt like he was the cause of the stress she was experiencing. The two of them sat down to enjoy the small spread he prepared.

So what's on the agenda for the remainder of the day? Sunny was asking because she was feeling horny but tired at the same time. The fruit that she was eating he was teasing Thaddeus with sexual antics.

"Stop playing beautiful, you're going to get into trouble." Thaddeus was telling Sunny. She wanted all the smoke.

Kissing one moment the next full blown out sex, the two had the oils from previous all over their bodies as Thaddeus made passionate love to Sunny. He began to confess his feelings for her and how excited he was to become a father with her as the mother of his child.

They went at it sex for another thirty minutes until both fell off to sleep in each other's arms.

Chapter 12

The morning at Majestic Massage Spa was quiet, ever since Thaddeus placed himself on a restricted schedule from being exposed to the sexual massages that he had thrown himself into. That was his way of self-healing using sex as a vice. Thaddues didn't want to continue on that path, since meeting Sunny.

Sam: Done! You owe me (smile emoji)

Magic: Thank You. Name it and I'll make it happen.

The text was what Thaddeus had been waiting on, he knew that showing up to help Melissa was the right thing to do. Their relationship was over two years off and on. When she stooped low to drug him to get him to sleep with her unprotected he knew that wasn't a good look he knew he couldn't trust her any longer. Thankful that he had Sam to get a Plan B concoction together to give to Melissa. So Thaddeus knew she was pregnant because he was keeping tabs on her. One of his clients worked at the doctor's office, where Melissa went to confirm her pregnancy. Rubbing his hands down his face Thaddeus was glad that he was two steps ahead of Melissa.

Walking back his client which was one of his last sensual massage Thaddeus liked what he saw, he knew that being a masseuse was a hard job. It wasn't hard but the temptations that came with it was. So many opportunities to be with women with permission and consent had been all too familiar for Thaddeus.

"Follow me, Ms. Green, right this way." He told his client who was exceptionally beautiful, she completed her assessment form and at the bottom it was what he didn't expect: she wanted to see him ejaculate. Now that wasn't something that he did on a regular basis in front of his clients unless it was a fetish of theirs. To see this he was not thrilled but the five-hundred-dollar service requested had to be fulfilled.

"So I'm going to get started with the oils first and began your massage, Ms. Green. Then towards the completion I can get you the final request." Thaddeus told her, as he reviewed the NDA she signed. Placing the lavender and sage oil on his client Thaddeus began to massage her body using the deep molding technique he learned from the convention that he went to. He did a thorough job as to Ms. Green had fell off to sleep during the session. In Thaddues mind he had to prepare himself for the final show. When he woke Ms. Green she was eager to see that Thaddeus was ready to show her his talents. With a few strokes and a few movements of his hand it wasn't long before he was ejaculating all over the towel in his hand. The smile that Ms. Green had on her face was priceless. She leaned over towards Thaddeus saying, "I'm sure you wife is pleased with what you do, I know I would be."

"Thank you Ms. Green, get dressed and you can check out up front." Thaddeus kept it short he didn't want to lead any of his clients on like what happened with him and Melissa.

Oh Mr. Magic, I see you changed up on us, one of his former clients was sitting out in the lobby. He had given Rodney his intense sensual sexual clients. The young lady that was speaking Thaddeus enjoyed her tricks, but she wasn't the type for him. She didn't fit the profile he would want to continue in a relationship with of any kind.

"Hi Sherry, I hope Mr. Rod is treating you nice." Thaddeus shot back at her with a smile to show he was somewhat concerned about having to pass her on to someone else.

"Oh yes, I wish I had rotated the two of you. Thank you for the referral." She stated as Rodney was coming back to help get her taken care of.

The day came to an end with all clients being seen and then new ones had scheduled an appointment with the team of Majestic Massage Spa. Sam was closing out the books when she saw Thaddeus heading to the breakroom.

"Thaddeus, I'm ready to collect my payment. I need a trip for two to Jamaica at the Sandals resort. If you can grant Charlie the time off, I'm taking her with me." Sam was looking at Thaddeus with a straight face. Laughing at the request, he looked at Sam then said, "You are serious aren't' you? Does she know you are requesting her presence on your little thotiana trip."

The two of them laughed. Thaddeus knew Charlie was bi-sexual. What he didn't know is that Sam was into that lifestyle too. It all made sense to him when he would come around them so they got quiet.

"So how long have you been sneaking around? Does Miles know you are a woman too?" with his eyebrow raised looking over at Sam.

"Well, no I hadn't broken it off with him yet. Me and Charlie have been getting to know one another big brother, so mind your business." Sam stated to Thaddeus.

"Okay, just book it and use the company card. You better not hurt Charlie either, she is special to me Sam. Matter of fact you both are special to me, so I'm watching you a little closer." Thaddeus told her just as Charlie came into the breakroom. Sam looked over at her with a smirk on her face, then blurted out.

"I told him, he knows now. So stop being all scary." She laughed at Charlie as she pulled her in for a kiss and pat on the behind.

"Oh hell, naw you too that's sexual harassment. I need to get the two of you to sign the NDA like the clients." Thaddeus was now looking on to both of them with a serious look.

"Really, says the man who has a woman trying to trap them, coming all on the job acting like a donkey. Going to your bae job acting like your dick made of crack." The three of them laughed, but Thaddeus wasn't laughing as hard. He was hurt that it came to those kinds of antics from a woman. The time he got hurt by a woman he knew it wasn't a good feeling. When you try to be cautious it sometimes doesn't work out that way.

"You to get out of here, I'm heading to see my baby momma." Thaddeus told them.

The night was clear as Sunny was preparing for her the next day. She had gotten a call from Thaddeus earlier today letting her know he was coming over after he finished work.

Thaddeus pulled into Sunny's driveway; he sat in his car for another twenty minutes reflecting back on all the happiness that had come into his life. The way his business was bombing even if he scaled back on the more intimate part, but the Majestic Massage Spa was rated in the top five for the city.

The drama with Melissa had seemed to die down, when she realized that Thaddeus was off limits as he told her in the beginning of the relationship.

"Hey, handsome," Sunny, spoke to Thaddeus as she let him into her home.

"Hey beautiful, how are you and the baby? You look great, still not showing as much." Sunny smiled as she felt the desire he has for her.

"Come in baby, I got a new fragrance I want you to try on me. It's pineapple sage, in a candle form. Once the wax melts you can rub it on me. Then I want you to do that trick with your fingers." Sunny was now blushing so hard from the thoughts of Thaddeus giving her a good massage with the new candles and oils she had purchased.

"Yes, let me set up the table so we can get started." He told her.

"No, let's go into my bedroom, it's more comfortable in there for me. I'm sure you will enjoy it better and so will I." that was all that he needed to hear. The two of them headed into Sunny's room so he could pleasure her the way she liked. "Baby, I have something for you too." She told him, smiling at him. Thaddeus was already semi hard from the thoughts of what he knew Sunny could do to him. The way she would suck and lick him from the back made him want to skip her and go straight to his part.

"Come on baby, before I ask for mine first." He said.

The music was turned on at a low volume in Sunny's room, she had already set the mood. Thaddeus was impressed by how Sunny set up her room to be a mini spa. The way she had towels ready, the oils and candles all around the room.

"What? Why are you standing there looking surprised? "Sunny was already dressed in a skimpy nightie under her little maxi dress. When she pulled the shoulders down, it was on. There wasn't anything left to the imagination under the maxi dress. Thaddeus was hard as Chinese arithmetic.

"Damn, baby! Come here I'm about to skip the massage then go to it later." He pulled her in for a passionate kiss, with his hands going all over her body. He pulled off her thongs as he put her on the bed, lifted her legs up to see what he claimed already as his. The move that he made landed him directly in the middle of her center. His delightful pleasure, he called it. Thaddeus began to lick and suck on Sunny's clit until she released it in his mouth multiple times. It wasn't a game for him; he loved the way she tasted from the first time he had her.

Oohhh, the moans that she released from her mouth caused him to sped up more and he continued sucking and licking on her. Thaddeus inserted two fingers and released a moan himself, "Baby, you are soaking wet," is this what I have to look forward to for the next few months. Arching her back Sunny welcomes whatever Thaddeus delivered to her. She was enjoying the moment releasing all the stress she had faced today. Although it was only phone calls and emails, she needed that release from the man she enjoyed it with. Sunny leaned her head back into the bed only to think of how happy she was. Thaddeus didn't give her any warning before she lifted his head up from being down onto her clit for a few minutes as he stood to enter into her. Normally he would ram his hard dick inside of her but today it had to be delicate. He would bust prematurely if he rammed it in due to how excited he was to feel her around him. Thaddeus was definitely in love with Sunny. The times with any other woman couldn't compare, even if he were using all his tricks from the class he took on pleasure and pleasing a woman.

"Sunny, baby I'm about to cum...." Was all Thaddeus could get out before he had already released himself deep inside of her. It was nothing for her to welcome all of his seeds due to the fact that she was already pregnant no damage could be done.

"Yes, baby," she responded into his ear. The two had to regain their breathing to continue on to the task at hand. Thaddeus got himself together quicker than Sunny, he lit the main candle so it could begin to melt he used the lavender and eucalyptus oils to start on her back and legs. When she stood for long periods of time she complained of cramps. So he made sure to work those areas first. Then he went down to her hips, the way he massage them made her want to gyrate on him. Thaddeus told Sunny, "Hey baby, you can't be doing that we got to get you taken care of. You are about to start something moving your hips like that."

Sunny wasn't thinking that she knew it was feeling so good that she continued without thinking of the consequence that would happen if she continued. Thaddeus continued as he worked the areas that Sunny was tense. Once he finished he used the pineapple sage wax pouring it on her body and she enjoyed it. The smell was so passionate he told her , "This is your scent baby, I love this on you." As he worked in the wax and it blended into her skin. Thaddeus was in heaven.

The next thirty minutes the two of them enjoyed the massage that Thadeus gave to Sunny. When it was her turn to return the pleasure Thaddeus couldn't handle it. Sunny introduced him to the pressure points of his body; she would bring him to ecstasy and he loved it.

"Lay back baby, stop trying to see what I'm doing." Sunny instructed him, she had become a pro at pleasing and pleasuring her man. Thaddeus loves every moment of it. What turned out to be his passion he found someone who loved it just as much as he did. Their relationship was more than just sex it was getting to know one another's likes and dislikes. That was what the two of them missed out in their previous relationships.

The next week Thaddeus and Sunny had planned to meet up to go over plans for the new life changes that were coming. He expressed the goal of new business ventures that included Sunny and the new addition. Sunny was happy that her business was able to be mobile, she had expressed adding more to her craft the introduction of exotic fragrances to the Spa.

Thaddeus suggested that they seek counseling too. That was his hidden secret, he had plans to make Sunny a permanent fixture in his life. The moment he realized that he loved her so much. With encouragement from their close circle their dreams would become a reality.

"Thaddeus, let's create a checklist so once we accomplish something we can check it off." Sunny suggested.

"Yes beautiful I agree, let's start with a quickie first." Thaddeus had that sex smile on his face, Sunny was all in. They made love like they owned the act, like they were the first to invent it. Passion was all over them. Later into the night Thaddeus just watched as Sunny slept. He was happy that he took the chance on her, that she didn't reject his advances in getting to know her.

Chapter 13

Six Months Later

Thaddeus was sure that the move to Vegas was best for his family, him Sunn and their beautiful daughter Thea. When he suggested the move Sunny didn't hesitate she was content with her position in his life. Their way of communicating was priceless. The thing was Thaddues appreciated she was a reality. She knew of his pessimistic ways, which didn't bother her. She was just as bad as he was always doing what she thought was for a good feeling. The one night stand she took a chance on with him changed both of their lives. Sunny's playlist consisted of the hottest hip hop artist with the hottest soundtracks that were out. She played every song that made her entire body jump as her soul moved to the beat. The way her vibe meshed with Thaddeus was the icing on the cake.

The song blasted out from the stereo as they unpacked their new home. It was ACT BAD, by the City Girls, which was Sunny's favorite or one of her favorites that she knew all the lyrics. While she sang the lyrics she danced around putting on a show for Thaddeus, he eased up behind her, "So you want to ACT BAD? Come on, show me."

Smiling really hard Sunny began to grind her hips until Thaddeus had her pinned up against the wall in their new home. Their little girl had already passed out from the excitement of a new place. She was asleep so the two did what they enjoyed exploring one another.

"Baby, when are you going to share your secret with me?" he asked Sunny, who wasn't sure what he meant from that statement.

"Huh, baby you are blowing the mood." Was her response.

"Okay, we will just go with the flow." Thaddeus said as he continued rubbing all over her body. The secret he knew was that Sunny was pregnant but not telling him that she was.

Kissing all over her body, every inch from her feet to her forehead. The moans that Sunny released were to his pleasure.

"Thaddeus baby ..... " She got out before her climax when he filled her up with his rock-hard penis. How could he ruin the goodness that he enjoyed with the woman that changed him.

The two shared multiple orgasms being delivered from each other. Upon the final one for the night the two passed out on the sofa that was still in the covered sheet from the move.

It was early AM a few days after Thaddeus and Sunny settled into a routine of living in a new city. He was handling his business as usual not working but two days or less a week. Allowing his income to come from both Spas. The investments he made and the speaking engagements he would do were comfortable. While opening his emails Thaddeus noticed one from Sam.

Dear Boss Man,

I would like to say thank you for being such a wonderful person, although you picked up and left us, HAHA we miss you so much. The paperwork came into day regarding the incident that happened with Melissa. She was found guilty, sentenced to eighteen months jail time, restitution of the damages and must complete a mental health course. Just wanted to let you know that issue was resolved. Enjoy yourself and take care of your beautiful family.

Sam, Charlie, and Rodney

Closing out his emails Thaddeus had a huge smile on his face. Sitting back in the chair he let out a huge sigh of relief. To have something they could control you wasn't what he wanted out of life, he didn't think that would be what anyone wanted out of life. Prior to Thaddeus meeting Sunny he was with Melissa in a non-committed relationship he was humping and pumping almost a half dozen women a month either meeting them outside of his work, or at his workplace. It was only a matter of time before it would catch up with him. Now that this issue was handled he could go on with his life as a normal person.

Looking up Thaddeus knew his wife was in the room, the fragrance she wore still did something to him. He smiled when he saw Sunny standing in front of him.

"Come her beautiful, what brings you in today?" he asked.

"I just wanted to run something by you, but not until we try out this new scent I picked up from the new candle shop I found." Sunny was big on candles and oils since being with Thaddeus anything to bring clients to grow their business. It was a new lavender scent that had a hint of flowers that she made up on her own.

"Nice, I like it," Thaddeus said as he poured the candle wax onto his skin. The wax wasn't too hot, it just fell on his skin to be rubbed on. Sunny was smiling as she told Thaddeus that her next concoction would be edible wax. That turned him on to the point that he was pulling Sunny's skirt up to devour her essences. It took no time for her to consent to his every move, allowing her man to taste her goodness; she then returned the pleasantries to him.

"Wait, baby I have a client in another hour. We can't," Thaddeus was trying to stop Sunny when she said, "Oh yes Sasha she will have to wait." With a raise of his brow Thaddeus was laughing now thinking that Sunny had a wonderful sense of humor.

"So you are Sasha," you little devil. "I knew it was something about that fact sheet, the things she was asking for we didn't even offer."

Thaddeus was shocked how Sunny had tried to play him; the fact sheet was asking for a serious happy ending. The ultimate massage from head to toe, sensual massage with a vaginal tantra. Sunny knew that he didn't do those anymore, and it was only done by the head masseuse in the spa, Max. When Max came to interview Thaddeus immediately knew he would be a good fit, he was every bit of a manly man. The full package.

"Come here woman, give me what you know I want." Thaddues told Sunny. She obeyed with her naked body now sitting on his lap, she easily opened up his pants to sit herself down with what was hers. Easing down she lifted herself up and down several times. When the final climax of the two happened they had to clean themselves up before they would be caught by their employees.

****

Thaddeus was heading home when he remembered that he had to pick up some things from the store. He called Sunny to make sure she didn't need anything, only to be told to bring back some ginger ale for her upset stomach. In his mind he knew he had been trying to get her pregnant again since it hadn't happened yet he was becoming frustrated. Taking the items into the house Thaddeus heard the music playing coming from their bedroom. Sunny was having a mini concert. First he stopped by his baby girl's room. Thea was a blessing to him. When she was born Thaddeus was the happiest man in the hospital that day. Sunny had an easy pregnancy and birth. Thea Sunni Kofi was born at seven pounds and four ounces, twenty inches long. Thaddeus was tall so he knew his baby girl may get his height, he just knew she would.

Sunny was singing her favorite hot girl summer jam by Sexy Red, Pound Town, she was dancing all over the room. Thaddeus had cracked the door halfway to get a clear view of his wife. Sunny had on just a skimpy red two-piece thong and bra set. Looking at her dance around singing every lyric was so funny to him. He got out his phone to record her for later.

Sunny was singing, my booty hole brown, as she bent over twerking to the beat. She blurted out I'm looking for a hoochie daddy, using her hands like she was looking around.

Still in a mood of singing and enjoying herself, Sunny didn't notice that Thaddeus had entered the room until she turned around doing a little bounce with her hips shaking.

"Oh so you looking for a hoochie daddy, huh?" he laughed as Sunny kept going on singing her song. The two of them were now sitting down as she continued to listen to her song.

Sunny told Thaddeus he was right a few nights ago. She had something she wanted to tell him.

"You bring my ginger ale?" she asked.

"Yes, I knew you weren't feeling well, for the last few weeks." He gave her a side eye.

"Well you are correct Mr. Thaddeus Kofi. While you were dicking me down you deposited your special seeds to make another little person. I'm pregnant." Sunny said without a blink of an eye, with a huge smile on her face.

Thaddues was smiling as he began to dance all around the room just as Sunny was doing when he arrived home. The two of them joined in with each other as the song was set on replay. Sunny led off with the lyrics she liked as loud as she could sing while Thaddeus just joined in on the hook only, Pound Town and he added his own twist

Pound Town you got dick down by a Masseuse, Pound Town just dicked you down.

They laughed at the antics that they created with each other. Thaddeus was so happy and so was Sunny. The two enjoyed each other and the storyline of how they got to this point.

"Come on baby, let me put those lyrics to work." Thaddeus pulled Sunny into his arms, giving her a passionate kiss. She just melted knowing that she enjoyed what he had to deliver. There was no resistance towards her man. The couple just sang for another thirty minutes while Sunny prepared for what Thaddeus was ready to deliver to her another round of real-life Pound Town.

Epilogue

Thaddeus was so happy at this time in his life having a second business open in the same location that he met the love of his life. Vegas gave him a sense of relief and a chance to restart his outlook on life. The name of his new shop really showed Majestic Sunshine Massage and Spa. When he pitched the idea to Sunny she was all in. It would be run by a team that was handpicked by the both of them. It was decorated by Sunny and brought a feel of calm as soon as you walked into the door. It had natural earth tones, beautiful décor that had you either in the desert or on the deep blue sea. They also offered the oils, bath salts, and other exotic massage props. The two of them were so happy to have thought of this idea.

Thaddeus was only doing massages twice a week. When Sunny had the baby he calmed down completely, he did most of the massages on her. His few clients understood but thanks to Rodney and Charlie they were pleased. Sunny, come on, we are going to miss the plane. Thaddeus was yelling out for Sunny to come on; they were late to the airport. It's been a year to be exact since the two of them met in Vegas. Now they had a one-year-old little girl Thea, she was the splitting image of Thaddeus with long thick black hair. It was as if Sunny didn't have anything to do in her features.

The two of them were headed to the AMT convention that was being held in Arizona this year. Thaddeus was being recognized for his business tactics of how to be prosperous in the industry. Everyone who was getting into the sensual and tantra massage looked to him to know how to handle the business. Since there was not much information on the ins and outs they looked to Thaddeus to give his expertise on the day-to-day process.

Sunny was happy to see that she fit right into his life, with her having her own business Thaddeus didn't take away her identity. She was like glue to him giving him some ideas to run a successful business.

"Look, baby, I don't want to leave without Thea, she is going to miss us." Sunny was stalling trying to convince Thaddeus one last time to bring their daughter to the convention.

"Sunny, we can't bring her, we won't get any work done. Plus, how will we be able to get her a brother or sister? She will be there looking at us and you know how she is with me." Thaddeus was being honest. Thea was spoiled rotten, knowing that he wouldn't be focused.

"Okay, since you put it like that." Sunny smiled at him.

"Lynn and Natalie will keep her company; she won't even miss us." Thaddeus was right Thea loved her cousins, just as much as her parents. Children will put you to the side when they know they can get what they want without any push back. Little Thea knew that early.

Once Thaddeus and Sunny arrived at the airport they had boarded the plane, the only thing was it wasn't heading to Arizona it was heading to Punta Cana DR. When the pilot announced the destination, Sunny looked up at Thaddeus.

"What did he say? Baby are we on the wrong plane." Sunny was now about to panic until she looked at her man. He was looking at her with a big smirk on his face. Pulling out his laptop he ignored Sunny's gaze when he powered on his laptop he turned it on to the video that he and his baby girl made. Showing it to Sunny he was waiting for her to respond.

"Mama, will you marry my daddy?" little Thea had worked hard on that spill and she did well. Thaddeus had been trying to get her to say it for about a month. When he realized that he was going to be honored at the convention he made a detour in the flight plans. They would go to the DR, get married and then return to Arizona in time for the last night of recognition to get his award.

Thaddeus had been planning the way he wanted to propose to Sunny for months. Teaching his baby girl how to say will you marry my momma to making all his travel plans for the stop to get married. He had already had her sign the marriage certificate with the help of her cousin Lynn. So once they got to DR the private beach wedding would be perfect for them. Thaddeus had planned everything down to the exact moment. When they arrive in the DR; the rest of the family will arrive two days later. Lynn was in on the plan to get their little girl and everyone else there. He was excited to have such a beautiful woman by his side.

"Sunny, I love you," Thaddeus expressed once Sunny accepted the proposal. She still didn't actually know the locations of her wedding. Relaxing on the plane as they continued on the journey happily ever after.

"Thaddeus you're full of surprises. The night we met I could never have thought this would lead to us. My goal was to get over the trails of life. Not thinking a hot steamy one-night stand would have us here. I love you Magic" she said with a devilish smile on her face.

The ride was smooth, when they landed in the DR, it was all five-star treatment. Thaddeus didn't hold back any stops. The resort staff met them at the airport with a luxury limo ride with fresh fruit and champagne for the ride. When they arrived they got the presidential suite with a beautiful ocean view. Sunny was in tears; she knew that this was real but still in disbelief.

"Sunny, get ready, we are going to the spa. "Thaddeus called out from the back of their room. "We have an appointment in another thirty minutes." She was surprised with the gesture.

Thaddeus had asked if he could have the spa for an hour, he wanted to show Sunny the time of her life. He had brought with him some of the oils and candles that they had created for one another. What Sunny didn't know he created a special fragrance for her only.

When he gave the instructions to the staff they were so happy to accommodate him.

Thaddeus pulled the door open for Sunny and she cried when she recognized the scents in the air. She knew it was personal for them, nobody had those oils, or scents but the Majestic Massage Spa. Her tears made Thaddeus happy since they were of joy.

"Baby, you didn't? How did you do this?" she asked.

"There is nothing I wouldn't do for you, my sunshine. Sunny, come on, you are going to enjoy this." Thaddeus was moving slowly towards the room that was assigned to them for hours. Once inside he escorted Sunny who was hands on, she had already taken her dress off and was pulling on Thaddeus pants. He was weak to her touch, not stopping her at all. He allowed her to take inside her mouth, who was he to stop his soon to be wife. The next ten minutes Sunny went to work giving Thaddeus all the pleasure he desired.

"Sunny baby I'm .... " he released down her throat without any hesitation just the way she liked. Sunny went to rinse out her mouth and was heading to the massage table. Thaddeus had lit a new scent with which she wasn't familiar. Sunny lifted a brow when he gave her the label of the new candle. It read Black Amour, it was the scent of the fragrance Black Love and Amber.

The couple was so engaged in the spa that they forgot about the time. Thaddeus began to end his massage on Sunny while the music played their favorite songs. When the Sexy Red track Pound Town came on they both began to sing the lyrics. Thaddeus wasn't thinking of how it was more of a song for women; he knew that he lived some of those lyrics. The best part was Sunny also enjoyed the lyrics to her favorite song for the summer as well.

Thankful for the trip they two enjoyed themselves the day the surprise wedding was at hand. Sunny was not happy that morning; she wasn't ready to leave the DR. Thaddeus told her that they would enjoy the resort to the fullest on the last day. He guided her to the spa again where they would have one last day.

"Sunny, come on, you're going to make us late." Thaddeus called out to her.

"I'm sad baby," she told him she wasn't ready to leave

Walking into the spa, Sunny was so surprised to see her cosine Lynn sitting in the waiting area. Her tears were enough to calm Thaddeus' nerves.

"What are you doing here?" Sunny asked, turning to look at her man. "You are so sneaky? Where is my baby?" just as Sunny asked out runs her little girl Thea who hugged her mommies legs.

The ladies were getting ready when Lynn asked for some advice from her cousin. Sunny was excited that her cousin had found love but ignored it. So when Lynn asked if she was happy with Thaddeus Sunny told her yes, it may seem fast but we are good together. Lynn was happy to hear that as she had her own dilemma with Thaddeus' cousin. "Lynn go with the flow, don't fight it. Look at me a few years ago I was not happy with my life. Now I'm doing what is right. Plenty sex, plenty of love with this little girl of mine, she is the bonus."

The four of them , Sunny, Thea, Lynn, and Natalie, also Sam, were pampered as they got ready for the wedding. In another part of the resort was Thaddeus, Nathan, Rodney, and Charlie. In less than thirty minutes the ceremony was to begin. It was such a beautiful beach front wedding that was full of love. The officiate pronounced the beautiful couple to the crowd. 'I now introduce to you Mr. and Mrs. Thaddeus Kofi."

It was cheered with clapping as the music blasted out to announce the newly married couple.

Congratulations was in order as they had a small reception. Sunny was glowing as Thaddeus snuggled up to her on the dance floor. He was whispering in her ear," You know you're pregnant right, I'm sure we made our son on this trip."

****

Sam walked into the Majestic Massage Spa with a frown on her face the building had been vandalized. The words that were spread over the outside windows read, SEX TRAP. It didn't make any sense to her; she took several photos of the windows then the broken glass sending it to Thaddeus.

"What is that? Call the police Sam." Thaddeus told her as he was heading into the office himself. "Don't go inside until they arrive. I'm about thirty minutes away.

Thaddeus got on the phone calling his security company to pull the tapes, then he asked for the ring camera footage that was on the outside of the building. He began to think who could have done something to damage his building or image.

"Hey Sam," Thaddeus called out asking her how she was knowing that she was upset when she arrived to open up the Spa.

"I'm all right the police are already inside; the forensics team is dusting for prints. You are going to have to brace yourself, they damaged your office the worse. It's personal Thaddeus," she was explaining to him what it looked like inside then froze at the sound of his phone notifications.

"Hold on, Sam I'm going to see for myself." Thaddeus took long strides inside to get to his office. "What the ....." his office was a complete mess, all his certificates were torn, the awards he received were broken. The piece to the puzzle was pictures of him and a woman whose face wasn't shown was plastered all over the walls thrown on the floor, Thaddeus knew who it was once he saw the pictures. He fell to the floor with his head down in his hands. Sam came into the office leaning down with him. She whispered into his ear, "Get up, this was pure hate, you are not in that place anymore. You have been healed from that painful place."

Sam was telling him the truth of what and how far he has come.

"Why?" Thaddeus cried out. "Sunny would be livid had she been with me to see this. I've been clean from that lifestyle for over a year." Thaddeus was in lite sobs.

"Hold your head up, let the law handle her, this was nothing but to get a response from you." Sam explained, "Let them handle it." Just as easy as Sam went on to let him know his worth she was also picking up the photos to place them in the shredder.

Buzz, Buzz, the notifications on his phone were going off. Checking to see who it was he had several text messages along with a few missed calls from Sunny. Opening his text messages, it was from his social media page he was tagged in with Sunny. The photos had been sent to their direct messenger. It was the same pictures, with Melissa's face plastered all over them.

Thaddeus wasn't impressed; he knew he had to call his wife immediately.

The phone was answered well before the first ring was completed. "Hello, Thaddeus are you alright?" Sunny's voice was calm.

"Baby, she vandalized the shop that is getting old Sunny." Thaddeus stated, "I apologize baby it wasn't meant to be like this."

Sunny listened as Thaddeus vented his emotions to her, when she thought he was finished she gave him the assurance he needed.

"Thaddeus, this is a cry for help for her. you haven't done anything wrong so don't let this worry you." Sunny stated. "Let the authorities handle it"

It was almost five hours before the forensics team had got all the prints they needed. The statement that Sam and Thaddeus gave helped to determine who was the person behind the damage to the building.

******

Life was too short to dwell on how past pain can cause you not to move forward in life. To have thought over the last year you could be only a few months to a positive loving further wasn't what both Thaddeus and Sunny had on the front of their mind. Now they have a new love for life and one another. It's easy to dwell on pain but much healthier to move forward in happiness, joy, and family.

I hope you enjoyed the story of two people taking that leap of fun excitement and plenty of sensual sexuality with a common goal of love. The active word that is easily defined with your heart if you allow it. Oh and yes Thaddeus didn't hit a homerun on the honeymoon but a few months later he did score with the implant of two seeds. They will be expecting twins in the future, who knows you might get to see them again in the story of their cousins Nathan and Lynn.